Healing Thyroid

Why You Still Have Thyroid Issues
And How To Fix Them

By

Neal Brown

Table of Contents

1. Introduction 5

2. Thyroid Gland Disorder Classifications 9
   Diseases due to Excessive Hormonal
   Secretion 9
   Diseases due to Diminished Hormonal
   Secretion 14
   Drug-induced Thyroid diseases 18
   Tumors of the Thyroid Gland 19

3. Hypothyroidism: Living in the slow lane 21
   Recognizing the Signs and Symptoms of
   Hypothyroidism 24
   Diagnosing Hypothyroidism 31
   Medical Treatment of Hypothyroidism 34

4. Natural Treatment of Hypothyroidism 44
   Hypothyroidism and a Gluten-free Diet 44
   Important Nutrients for Thyroid 46
   The Role of Tyrosine 51
   The Role of Vitamins 52
   The Role of Balanced Free Fatty Acids 54

    Dietary goitrogens 56

    Thyroid Supplements 57

    The Autoimmune Protocol Diet 61

    Lifestyle Changes for Hypothyroidism 63

5. Hyperthyroidism: I'm a Ferrari! 67

    Recognizing the Signs and Symptoms of Hyperthyroidism 69

    Diagnosing Hyperthyroidism 76

    Medical Treatment of Hyperthyroidism 78

    Natural Treatment of Hyperthyroidism 88

    Which Foods to Include in Diet 101

    Lifestyle Changes for Hyperthyroidism 108

6. A Guide to Thyroid Tests 112

    Blood Tests 112

    Radioactive Iodine Tests 117

    Specific Tests for Hypothyroidism 119

7. Shopping: An Add-to-Cart Kindda Day 124

    Fruit & Vegetables 124

    Alternatives to Dairy/Milk 125

    Animal Products 125

    Nuts & Seeds 126

Pasta, Rice & Grains	126
Fats and Oils	127
Tinned/Bottled Foods	127
Beans	128
Condiments & Spices	128
8. Conclusion: Remembering What it is Like to Feel Normal	**129**
References	131
Disclaimer	149

1. Introduction

Every day, you grab your keys, sit in the car and twist the ignition key. A little spark of electricity ignites in every cylinder of the engine and before you know it, you are out on the road and driving towards your destination. Now consider having a car with an eight-cylinder capacity but only with seven spark plugs in a working state. Your car will not stop running but it will definitely run roughly.

Inside your body, the thyroid hormone functions exactly similar to that of a spark plug. It ignites your body, releases the stored energy and drives the cellar reactions which allow your body to hum along. So, what will happen if your thyroid starts losing its spark someday?

It is quite possible that you may be among the 59 million U.S. citizens experiencing the mysterious and more importantly, the undiagnosed symptoms of a malfunctioning thyroid gland. Even if you are lucky enough to get a proper diagnosis, there is a lot more to deal with.

Let's suppose your doctor diagnoses you with a thyroid issue. It will take a couple of years for your labs to finally catch up. If you are lucky enough, you may be prescribed the magic pills but if you don't, you will opt for every natural way to a healthy thyroid. You will make a quick search on the internet, note down the things to eat, work out every day, and wake up feeling refreshed one day.

Sounds easy, right? This is not how it is going to turn out for you.

Imagine yourself fighting with the dreadful symptoms of a malfunctioning thyroid gland, continuously finding your way to treat it naturally, while some glowing beauty arrives and hands you a green-colored juice with ginger, kale, cucumber, and lime. You take it and suck it up only to find it revitalizing every cell of your body.

Green juice becomes a normal part of your routine and you finally start feeling invigorated until you come across some food blog that blasts the news of avoiding green veggies especially if you are suffering from a thyroid issue.

This is probably going to make you think, "WHAT?" How can these veggies be bad for your thyroid when they were making you feel revived and full of energy?

As you continue reading the blog, you come across various contraindications. Eat more broccoli, munch on spinach and consume kale to increase glutathione and make thyroid healthy. That's when you are confused. You push the green juice away and start eating a gluten-filled sandwich because you are feeling sorry for yourself. The blogs told you to avoid gluten, but you just aren't sure anymore.

We firmly believe that any thyroid issue is not a one-size-fits-all type of condition and it is most definitely not easy to treat. That is why this book brings you a wealth of information about thyroid, its biology, diagnostic tests, and treatment options, all of which helps you to gradually understand the difference between a good and a bad treatment option. It is much more than a cookery book or a pharmaceutical directory for thyroid drugs. In fact, the book is a step-by-step manual for every reader who wants to understand thyroid issues and the ways to resolve them.

2. Thyroid Gland Disorder Classifications

When the thyroid gland is working at a normal pace, it secretes two principle hormones, T3 or triiodothyronine, and T4 or thyroxine.[1] In a malfunctioning thyroid, the concentration of these hormones becomes abnormal depending on the type of disorder. The disorders of the thyroid can be broadly classified into different categories, particularly depending upon the causative factors.[2]

Diseases due to Excessive Hormonal Secretion

Having too much thyroid hormone, a condition known as hyperthyroidism is one of the basic categories of thyroid gland disorders. This can be due to a number of factors such as Grave's disease, nodules on the thyroid, infection, or even drugs.

Graves' Disease

It is common to confuse hyperthyroidism, which means an overactive thyroid gland, and Graves' disease, which refers to a condition in which there is excessive thyroid hormone in the body. These two conditions can be regarded as cousins that may be able to pass as twins.[3]

All the "hypertrophied" signs and symptoms that you have heard about are actually related to having too much thyroid hormones in your body which may be a consequence of an overactive thyroid. However, this does not mean that hyperthyroidism is the sole cause of Graves' disease.[4] Graves' disease may occur due to a lot of other reasons.

Grave's disease is an autoimmune disorder of the thyroid which clinically presents with hyperthyroidism. Autoimmune diseases develop when your body's own immune system starts attacking the healthy tissues. The primary mechanism of autoimmunity is not completely understood so far, however, a genetic connection seems to be prevalent, espexcially in case of Graves' disease.[5] Just like most of the autoimmune disorders, Graves' disease also affects women more than men.[6]

In Grave's disease, the immune system produces antibodies that force thyroid to grow in size and increase its hormone production. These autoantibodies, known as thyroid-stimulating immunoglobulins or TSIs, attack themselves to the receptors for thyroid-stimulating hormone (TSH); a hormone that regulates the thyroid for hormone production. In this way, the TSIs trick the thyroid into believing that the body needs more hormones and hyperthyroidism occurs eventually. [7]

Multinodular Goiter

Another common reason for hyperthyroidism is a multinodular goiter. A goiter refers to a condition in which whole of the thyroid gland is evenly enlarged.[8] In contrast, a multinodular goiter is when multiple nodules appear on its surface. A multinodular goiter may or may not affect the hormonal production. If the autonomous nodules present on the thyroid are capable of causing hyperthyroidism, such type of goiter is what you know as toxic multinodular goiter.[9] Multinodular goiter is the second commonest cause of hyperthyroidism, secondary to Graves's disease.[10]

Multinodular goiter usually occurs due to a subsequent hypothyroidism. When your body is not making sufficient level of thyroid hormone, the pituitary gland present in the brain will release more TSH. High levels of TSH will keep acting on the thyroid giving rise to different nodules on it.

TSH-Producing Adenomas

Sometimes, the cause of hyperthyroidism lies in the brain, a condition known as secondary hyperthyroidism. The pituitary gland is an important part of the endocrine system that controls all the glands within a human body. As mentioned before, it produces called TSH which is responsible for regulating the functions of the thyroid.

TSH-secreting pituitary adenomas may be a reason why your thyroid hormone levels are elevated.[11] These are benign tumors that produce too much TSH. This increases the size of thyroid and forces it to work at a faster pace.

The patients with TSH-secreting adenomas of the pituitary glands suffer from the usual symptoms of hyperthyroidism. However, there may be some additional manifestations such as loss of visual field and constant headaches.[12]

Diseases due to Diminished Hormonal Secretion

Hypothyroidism is a state in which there is too little circulating thyroid hormone in your blood. It results from a thyroid that is incapable of producing sufficient hormone. It can occur due to radioactive ablation, nutritional deficiencies, atrophy, or an infection.

Sometimes, the treatment for certain hyperactive thyroid disorders like Graves' disease requires the removal of all or some part of this gland. In such circumstances, a vast number of patients become hypothyroid.[13]

Hashimoto Thyroiditis

Thyroiditis is the inflammation of thyroid gland. There are different types of thyroiditis, most common of which is Hashimoto's thyroiditis. Just like Graves' disease, Hashimoto's thyroiditis is an autoimmune disorder. It involves the aggravation of the immune system against the body's own tissues.[14]

In case of Hashimoto's thyroiditis, the body produces specific auto-antibodies that target the thyroid tissue causing irreversible damage. Since the thyroid becomes partially or completely damaged, it is unable to meet the body's normal requirements of thyroid hormones.[15] The levels of T4 falls in blood urging the pituitary to increase the levels of TSH for compensation.

Other types of thyroiditis include De Quervain's thyroiditis which follows a viral infection. It involves the generation of granulomas on the thyroid. If a bacterium attacks the thyroid and forms abscesses on it, it is known as acute suppurative thyroiditis.[16]

Secondary Hypothyroidism

Just like hyperthyroidism, the root cause of hypothyroidism may also lie outside the thyroid. This is known as secondary hypothyroidism and usually involves an abnormality in the brain. Secondary hypothyroidism is due to the disorders of the hypothalamus or pituitary gland. It is generally associated with a low level of T3, T4, or TSH hormones.

In some cases, the TSH levels seem to be normal despite the presence of secondary hypothyroidism. This makes TSH an unreliable tool for detection of the condition and must not be utilized for diagnosis. There can be a lot of causes of secondary hypothyroidism. The destruction of the pituitary gland or hypothalamus due to any inflammation, neoplasm, autoimmunity, or avascular necrosis may be the contributing factors.[17] There are a number of risk factors that make an individual prone to secondary hypothyroidism. The condition particularly hits people above the age of 50 and is more prevalent in females. Having a past medical history of pituitary or hypothalamus malfunction can also be a contributing factor.[18]

Peripheral Resistance to Thyroid Hormones

Sometimes, the cause of hypothyroidism is more complex than the malfunctioning thyroid or pituitary. Thyroid hormone resistance, also known as Refetoff syndrome, is a rare condition in which the thyroid hormone levels are elevated but no suppression of the TSH hormone occurs as expected in a normal condition.[19]

Mutations in the thyroid receptors are thought to contribute to Refetoff syndrome. The body tissues fail to respond to thyroid hormone and produce a condition of hypothyroidism despite having these hormones in normal amounts.

Drug-induced Thyroid diseases

Drug-induced thyroid diseases have a vast sub-categorization including diseases with hyperthyroidism, hypothyroidism, and even thyroiditis. Different drugs affect the thyroid differently and may or may not alter its hormone production.[20]

Amiodarone is a drug rich in iodine which is widely used for managing ventricular and atrial arrhythmias. This drug has a potency to interact with thyroid hormone metabolism and produce subsequent effects. Most of the patients consuming amiodarone remain euthyroid i.e. they do not produce any symptoms related to thyroid. However, some of them may develop hypothyroidism or Graves's disease.[21]

Another common offender in this respect is lithium, a medication used for treating the patients with bipolar disorders. Lithium works by reducing the abnormal brain activity and may also be prescribed for depression, blood disorders, and schizophrenia. At the same time, this drug has an ability to induce hypothyroidism in people, especially those with a pre-existing undiagnosed thyroid problem.[22]

Interferon alpha, a popular drug of choice for hepatitis C may cause the thyroid to inflame, leading to thyroiditis. Thyroiditis can also be caused by Interleukin-2, a medicine used for boosting immunity during cancer therapy.[23]

Tumors of the Thyroid Gland

The thyroid gland is made up of two major types of cells i.e. the follicular cells and C-cells. Other less important cells include stromal cells and immune cells. Each type of cells has a tendency to start growing at an abnormally high pace giving rise to tumors.[24]

Thyroid tumors are of two types; the benign tumors or thyroid adenomas are less dangerous as they do not have the potential to metastasize to other parts. Malignant tumors of the thyroid, also known as thyroid cancer, are further divided into follicular, papillary, anaplastic, and medullary types and are extremely dangerous.[25]

These tumors can invade the substance of thyroid and destroy the tissue leading to hypothyroidism. In some cases such as toxic multinodular goiter, the tumor may start producing thyroid hormones and set the stage for a hyperthyroid body.

3. Hypothyroidism: Living in the slow lane

By now, you are aware that the thyroid hormones keep your body functioning at the optimal speed. If these hormones decrease to a level below what is set as a normal point, the condition that prevails is hypothyroidism. Hypothyroidism slows down your body, signaling all the cells of the body to literally become lazy. As a consequence, a lot of organ systems start losing functionality and focus giving rise to a set of symptoms such as depression, excessive fatigue, skin dryness constipation, and weight gain.[26]

Most of the people are unable to connect the dots in favor of a thyroid disease. Almost ten million people suffer from hypothyroidism and it is said that a significant portion of them do not even know that they have it. In the year 2000, different blood tests were performed on almost twenty-six thousand random people visiting a statewide fair held in

Colorado. The researchers were amazed to find that about 10 percent of these tests indicated an elevated level of TSH suggestive of an undiagnosed hypothyroidism.[27]

Did you know that hypothyroidism has a tendency to hit more than one out of every eight women who have crossed the age of 50?

Even the ratio is so high in the older adults, the disease is least recognized in this age-group. This is because most of the symptoms of hypothyroidism seems to be more elusive in them. People over the age of sixty are less likely to manifest the classical symptoms of a thyroid disease as compared to the younger patients. In some cases, they only have one symptom, like depression or memory loss, both of which can be considered as signs of aging. In older females who do manifest the classic symptoms of fatigue and weight gain, these symptoms are mixed with the signs of middle age. [28]

This means that the physicians need to keep a higher index of suspicion to timely diagnose hypothyroidism, especially in older adults. Blood tests are the only tests which may confirm if you have hypothyroidism or not. So, it is imperative that you are fully aware of its symptoms and ask your healthcare for a complete thyroid evaluation if you have just crossed sixty, manifest the symptoms of hypothyroidism, or are included in the high-risk groups.

Thyroid tests are not a part of the routine assessment. They are not performed unless your physician has a solid reason to believe that you are symptomatic or are included in a high-risk group. If left untreated, a hypothyroid state can seriously affect your health with time. It can increase your risk for hypertension, hypercholesterolemia, and atherosclerosis. All of these conditions eventually put you at an elevated risk for cardiovascular complications such as a heart attack. With time, hypothyroidism develops into another condition called myxedema in which the body functions start slowing down to a dangerously low point, increasing the risk of coma.[29]

Recognizing the Signs and Symptoms of Hypothyroidism

As discussed earlier, the symptoms of hypothyroidism are highly variable making it extremely difficult for diagnosis. If you make two people suffering from the same disease stand side by side, you will notice that they will have entirely different sets of symptoms. One of them may have developed hypothyroidism in a matter of months, while the other took years to finally manifest it. Generally speaking, the lower the levels of thyroid hormone, the more symptoms will manifest. Sometimes, mild forms of hypothyroidism progress into more severe states, while in some cases, this does not happen. These anomalies are more pronounced in the patients of older age. If you are experiencing any of the following symptoms, have a doctor examine your thyroid.[30]

Fatigue

If your body is making the lesser concentration of thyroid hormone, less energy will be produced. This manifests itself in the form of extreme exhaustion. Some people feel like sleeping all day even if they have taken a good night sleep the previous night.

Chilly Feels

As the deficiency of thyroid hormone slows down your cells, they require a lesser amount of energy. Therefore, the total production of heat in your body falls drastically. If you have a malfunctioning thyroid, you will notice that you are the one who is turning up the heat even when the others are perfectly comfortable. You become highly intolerant to cold weather and require additional layers of clothing than the people surrounding you.

Loss of Appetite

Since your total energy requirements are decreased, the body craves for lesser calories. So, your appetite is naturally suppressed. Despite the fact that you are eating less, hypothyroidism may make you gain weight. At the same time, it gets really difficult for you to shed it even though you are eating a lot less than the usual.

Decreased Heart Rate

If you are a patient with hypothyroidism, you will definitely notice a difference in your heart rate. This difference is only detectable when you take your pulse. Low levels of circulating thyroid hormone can slow down the heart functioning and may even induce bradycardia. The usual heart rate in such patients falls below 60 beats per minutes.

Excessive Weight Gain

It is quite normal for a patient with hypothyroidism to gain weight. Even though you are eating much lesser than before, you are still consuming calories in an amount higher than what your body can metabolize. This is because low thyroid hormone has already slowed down the metabolic activities throughout your body and is currently converting calories into energy at an extremely slow rate.

Additionally, weight gain also occurs due to fluid retention in some cases. It is important to realize that while hypothyroidism makes you put on some extra pounds, it does not cause obesity.

Thyroid Enlargement

Even though the thyroid is underworking, it has a tendency to enlarge. This is true particularly when iodine deficiency or Hashimoto's thyroiditis is the causative factor of hypothyroidism.

Depression

The characteristics of hypothyroidism match closely to those of depression. Weight gain, reduced appetite, and fatigue are commonly observed in the patients with depression. Some patients with hypothyroidism even suffer from a perpetual state of dysphoria which can be clinically mistaken as depression. It is not unusual for a doctor to suggest antidepressants to a patient with an underactive thyroid. Hypothyroidism makes it difficult for you to concentrate and even lead to memory loss. You find yourself caring less about what is usually important for you. Studies have even estimated that autoimmune thyroiditis has a tendency to occur in about 20 percent of the people suffering from clinical depression as compared to only 5-10 percent of the normal population.

Skin Dryness

The sweat glands distributed in different parts of your body are responsible for keeping your skin hydrated. But when your body reduces its total heat production, you tend to sweat less. This reduces the activity of sweat glands and causes the skin to become dry. In chronic hypothyroidism, the skin also starts flaking off. Cracked skin is particularly visible around knees and elbows. Additionally, the fingernails become extremely brittle and their grooves become rough.

Hair Loss

Patchy hair loss is a common symptom of hypothyroidism. In some conditions, you may even start losing the body hair.

Constipation

Because hypothyroidism slows down your metabolic rate, the digestive processes start lagging behind. This causes constipation; dry, hard stools are passed out along with painful cramps that may be relieved by a bowel movement.

Vague Pains

Your body suddenly starts experiencing pain in muscles and joints that closely resemble the type of pain occurring in rheumatoid arthritis.

Menstrual Abnormalities

If you are a young female, hypothyroidism may cause your periods to occur more frequently. They also become heavier and cause changes in your ovulatory cycle. Hypothyroidism can even reduce a female's ability to conceive.

High Cholesterol

An underactive thyroid can cause your blood cholesterol to rise. Thyroid hormone assists the liver in forming the LDL receptors. As their level falls, fewer receptors for LDL are produced. This means that there are fewer molecules that pull out the LDL or bad cholesterol from the blood.

Carpal Tunnel Syndrome

A lot of people relate carpal tunnel syndrome with certain activities such as using the keyboard of a computer for long. However, this condition mostly accompanies certain diseases, hypothyroidism being one of them. If you suffer from carpal tunnel syndrome, you may feel tingling in your fingers and wrists. This is because the soft tissues in these areas along with the supporting ligaments swell up and compress the nearby median nerve.

Diagnosing Hypothyroidism

When must you have a thyroid test? According to the American Thyroid Association, all adults must be a screen for thyroid issues at the age of thirty-five years. The tests must take place regularly with an interval of five years. However, there seems to be a disagreement in the medical community regarding the cost-effectiveness of thyroid screening. So, your doctor may or may not routinely screen you for thyroid issues. You may not be recommended one even if you are gaining weight like crazy or feeling really tired all of a sudden because such symptoms are commonly experienced by a lot of problems and may be indicative of a broad spectrum of diseases. This is why it is easy for people with hypothyroidism to slip through the cracks.

To detect a case of hypothyroidism, it is best to ask your doctor for a thyroid checkup if you are thirty-five and above, or you are exhibiting any symptoms suggestive of a thyroid malfunction. Most of the time, the primary health care workers can easily treat hypothyroidism. However, certain conditions require the consultation or even a referral to an endocrinologist, a physician that has specialized in treating the disorders of hormones and glands. You may even require the consultation of a thyroidologist for more specific treatment. You may be asked to consult a specialist if you:

- Are pregnant

- Are a heart patient
- Suffer from a thyroid nodule or goiter
- Are under the age of eighteen
- Suffer from a coexisting problem

A test that can measure the levels of TSH in the blood is the best way to detect a thyroid problem. Additionally, a doctor may like to check the size of your thyroid gland by palpating your neck area. It is also common to look for other physical manifestations of hypothyroidism such as hair loss, coarseness of hair, and skin dryness. All the nerve reflexes are checked in addition to assessing blood pressure and cholesterol levels.

If the amount of TSH in blood is abnormally high, a test for determining T4 levels is performed. If it comes out to be low, the condition is suggestive of hypothyroidism. To confirm the cause of hypothyroidism, the doctor may run some blood tests to detect the presence of antibodies.[31]

Medical Treatment of Hypothyroidism

If you have been tested positive for hypothyroidism, do not worry. Treatment for hypothyroidism exists without any peculiar complications. In the meantime, you can be happy putting a name to what has been making you miserable for and long time and to know that this condition can be managed.

A doctor is likely to prescribe a medication that replaces the missing thyroid hormone in your body. The goal of this hormone replacement therapy is to replicate the normal activity of the thyroid. The most commonly used agent is levothyroxine sodium, a pure synthetic form of thyroxine that works similar to that of your body's won thyroid hormone.[32]

If the doctor says that your condition is permanent, you might have to continue taking this medicine for the entire life. Some suggest that this is only a small sacrifice compared to the drastic adversities that hypothyroidism would cause otherwise. Levothyroxine sodium can dramatically improve your functioning once it restores the levels of thyroid hormones in the blood. You can keep hypothyroidism in control with just one dose of this drug every day. Additionally, there are no restrictions on diet and no lifestyle modification is usually required.

Because synthetic thyroid hormone is just a replacement for the naturally produced hormones in your body, the chances of side effects or any allergic reactions are little. If you suffer from goiter secondary to Hashimoto's thyroiditis, this synthetic hormone may be able to shrink it and prevent its recurrence.

How to Determine Your Dose

The initial dosage regimen for levothyroxine sodium requires careful analysis of several factors such as your age, weight, and any coexisting diseases.

Generally speaking, it is a rule to provide 1.7 mcg thyroid hormone for every kg of your body. Your physician may settle for a higher or lower dose according to your specific conditions.[33]

If you are older, the treatment will be gradual because of an elevated risk of a cardiovascular disease. Pursuing a full hormone replacement therapy too quickly can put a load on your heart and the central nervous system. On the other hand, managing it gradually allows both the brain and the heart to adjust themselves accordingly. For example, your physician may decide to start the therapy with 12.5 to 25 mcg of levothyroxine sodium per day. The dose gets increased every four weeks until the lab tests reveal that your blood levels of T4 and TSH have crossed the normal range. As you achieve a normal level of thyroid hormone, your doctor changes the schedule to an even more gradual pattern especially for those who suffer from angina, heart failure, or anxiety.

The dose also depends upon the severity of hypothyroidism in a patient. For example, if you suffer from autoimmune hypothyroidism, your body only requires partial replacement. This is because the thyroid is intact and working properly. However, if the underlying hypothyroidism is due to thyroidectomy i.e. the surgical removal of the thyroid gland, a complete hormonal replacement may be indicated with a higher dose of levothyroxine sodium. In the patients with cancer, a higher dose is recommended as it reduces the chances of recurrence.

Another important thing to consider while determining the dose is whether you are already taking any medication that may interfere with the thyroid drug. For example, if you taking an estrogen therapy, birth control pills, or specific antidepressants, you may require a relatively higher dose of levothyroxine sodium. Therefore, it is essential that you inform your doctor about any other medicines that you are taking at the moment before starting thyroid hormone replacement therapy.

Consider the initial dose as an experimental number. There is certainly a possibility of trial and error, mainly because your thyroid needs are quite precise and will require constant adjustments until the level of TSH in your body gets normalized. The doctor will begin with the minimal dose because too much of synthetic thyroid hormone can cause hyperthyroid symptoms like anxiety, tachycardia, or nervousness. If you suffer from any of these symptoms after commencing the therapy, inform your doctor immediately.

After settling on an initial dose, your body will require a few weeks to produce any changes in the system. Thyroxine has a slow mechanism of action; therefore, you may not feel its effects right away. The doctor will look for the TSH levels six to eight weeks after the initiation of the therapy to make dose adjustments. If the level of TSH has not been normalized, the doctor will keep making the necessary adjustments until it falls within the normal range. Once you have reached an appropriate dose, a test for TSH and free thyroxine will be performed every six months as a follow-up.

Levothyroxine vs Desiccated Thyroid

The most common treatment for hypothyroidism is levothyroxine which is a synthetic form of T4 hormone. It is known to be the most effective type of thyroid hormone which is extremely safe for the body. However, certain unwanted side effects are commonly reported including heat intolerance, fever, dysphagia, and irritability.[34] A few studies have also indicated that the chronic use of levothyroxine in a dose higher than 150 mcg per day can elevate the risk of osteoporosis in later stages of life. These side effects led the scientists to turn towards an alternative agent i.e. the desiccated thyroid.[35]

The desiccated thyroid, or Armour, is actually a mixture of T3 and T4 hormones and is said to be equally effective as levothyroxine. The clinical trials that used a mixture of T3 and T4 hormones have concluded that it can work just like levothyroxine for replacing thyroid hormone in the blood. In some cases, it has even surpassed its efficacy. This is why desiccated thyroid is often considered as a backup option for the patients who are unable to tolerate levothyroxine therapy.[36, 37,38]

It is important to know that certain types of desiccated thyroid are not regulated tightly in terms of quality or dose. Even though they require FDA regulation supplements do not usually have to pass through the same requirements for efficacy and safety as that for other pharmaceutical drugs.[39] In fact, a study has revealed that desiccated thyroid of more than half of the brands contain lower levels of T4. One particular variant was found to have no T4 at all. In simpler words, the use of desiccated thyroid has its own risks and no added benefit as compared to the standard therapy involving levothyroxine.[40] The only advantage of desiccated thyroid is that it is better tolerated. For deciding which medicine is better, you need to work with your doctor to discuss pros and cons of both. Only then can you come up with an answer which is best suited to your individual needs.

When to Take Thyroid Medicine

Thyroid hormone must be preferably taken on an empty stomach. This means you can take it every morning before breakfast, or at night before going to bed. You may also take it one hour outside of your meal times. This is important because food or beverage of any kind can reduce the T4 absorption in your body. This effect is particularly enhanced if you consume soy, coffee, or food rich in calcium, iron, and fiber. Dairy food, fruits, nuts, eggs, and meat can also interfere with the absorption of T4 so, just to be on the safe side, it is recommended to wait 2 hours instead of 1.[41]

Should you take thyroid medicine in the morning or at night? Many clinical trials have been held to investigate the most appropriate time for taking levothyroxine. Some of these studies have concluded that it is better to take the medicine in the morning whereas others state that the medicine works best when taken at night.[42,43] Many other trials found that the time of consumption held no importance in terms of efficacy. The inconsistencies in the results might be due to the variable dietary patterns and the nationalities of participants.[44,45] As it has been mentioned before that different types of food affects thyroid drug absorption differently. So, neither option can be regarded as better than the other.

If you wish to take your medicine in the morning, prefer taking breakfast later during the day. Alternatively, you may even skip the breakfast if you do not absolutely need it to begin the day. Opposing the popular beliefs breakfast is not essential for maintenance of good health. If you like to take it at night, avoid taking any food or beverage after 8 pm. Taking levothyroxine at night, however, causes insomnia in some of the patients and may also increase the urgency to urinate, so keep this in mind before choosing the most suitable time.

4. Natural Treatment of Hypothyroidism

Even though medical treatment has been fairly successful in managing hypothyroidism, a lot of people still prefer adopting the natural ways. For those, there are different ways to achieve a healthy thyroid.

Hypothyroidism and a Gluten-free Diet

Gluten is a type of protein that naturally occurs in wheat and grain. About 6 percent of the population is unable to digest it properly, and several studies have indicated a strong connection between hypothyroidism and what you know as gluten sensitivity or celiac disease. More than 18 percent of the people who suffer from celiac disease form antibodies that particularly attack the thyroid. It is important to remember that Hashimoto's thyroiditis also has a similar mechanism in which your immune system starts attacking the thyroid. Following this link, it can be said that a patient of Hashimoto's thyroiditis may benefit from a gluten-free diet, but does research support it?

Many studies have reported that consumption of a gluten-free diet decreases the total number of anti-thyroid antibodies. This signifies that the number of antibodies which target the thyroid can be reduced if gluten is avoided altogether.[46, 47] But before you stop reading this and divert all your energy in finding the perfect gluten-free recipes, it is important that you know that certain trials have not reported any improvements in hypothyroid patients even if they followed a gluten-free diet. The truth is that the scientists are yet to know the actual influence of gluten on hypothyroidism. For a regular person, however, there is no harm in trying out a diet free of gluten for a month and then assessing the status. These foods do not hold any unique nutritious value anyways.

Important Nutrients for Thyroid

Your eating pattern greatly influences the thyroid health. This is why it is crucial to develop an understanding of the key nutrients required for reversing an underactive thyroid.

1. Iodine

Iodine is a natural trace element of your body. It is required by the thyroid gland to produce its hormones. For this very reason, iodine deficiency may disrupt the thyroid function. However, this is seldom the cause of hypothyroidism, particularly in the developed countries where food is available in surplus amounts.

According to the World Health Organization (WHO), a person is rendered as an iodine deficient if his urine has less than 100 micrograms of iodine per liter. In the year 2003-04, the urine levels of iodine in Americans were recorded to be 160 micrograms per liter whereas, in Australians, the levels were 124 micrograms per liter.[48] To reduce the prevalence of hypothyroidism, more than a hundred countries made iodization of bread and salt mandatory. Although not mandatory in the United States, nearly half of the salt available in this country has iodine added to it. [49]

Nevertheless, the inclusion of foods rich in iodine can be safe for your thyroid. Some of these food sources include:

- Potatoes
- Cow's milk
- Navy beans
- Iodized salt
- Seafood
- Eggs

Remember that some of you may have a sensitivity to extra iodine. Moreover, consuming concentrated forms of iodine such as kelp tablets or iodine drops can worsen your thyroid and must not be consumed before consulting a doctor. Your optimal target must be to consume 150 mcg of iodine per day for replenishing the deficient levels.

2. Selenium

You may not know it but your thyroid requires selenium for recycling iodine. This is the reason why thyroid consists of the highest level of selenium of all the other body organs. It is logical to think that selenium deficiency can cause hypothyroidism via certain pathways that relate it to iodine.[50] For this purpose, it is necessary that you eat a diet rich in selenium. Some examples of selenium-rich food items include:

- Sardines
- Tuna
- Eggs
- Brazil nut
- Legumes
- Chicken and beef

The recommended dose for selenium in case of Hashimoto's thyroiditis and other types of hypothyroidism is 55 micrograms per day.

3. Zinc

The role of zinc in regulation of thyroid hormone is crucial. The metabolisms of both these agents are so closely linked that a deficiency may lead to loss of hair, a condition recognized by the healthcare workers as alopecia. [51] Although zinc deficiency is rather uncommon in the developed countries, it is safe to consume the following foods for getting an additional amount of zinc:

- Legumes
- Chicken and beef
- Oysters
- Seeds and nuts
- Yogurt and milk
- Shellfish

If a suspected zinc deficiency is causing hypothyroidism, consider taking 30 to 60 mg of this nutrient every day in your diet.

4. Iron

You must be aware of the role of iron in delivering oxygen to every cell of human body. This obviously includes your thyroid cells as well. Iron, along with many other minerals, is also essential for the synthesis of thyroid hormone.[52] Even though the role of selenium is bigger, the presence of iron is also necessary to carry out certain steps. Iron also helps in optimal functioning of the immune system which is particularly important for the patients of Hashimoto's thyroiditis.

Remember that people suffering from autoimmune thyroid issues commonly suffer from hypochlorhydria i.e. reduction of the total hydrochloric acid production in the digestive tract. This condition can particularly interfere with iron absorption and may lead to a subsequent deficiency. To naturally supplement your body with iron, consider eating the following foods:

- Eggs
- Meat
- Seeds and nuts
- Pulses
- Iron-fortified bread and cereals
- Soybeans
- Whole grains

The recommended dietary allowance for iron in adult males is 8mg whereas in females is 18 mg.

The Role of Tyrosine

Tyrosine is a naturally occurring amino acid that is necessary for the production of T4 thyroid hormone. Within an epithelial cell of the thyroid, iodide transforms into iodine which then incorporates itself into a tyrosine residue known as thyroglobulin. This combination of iodine and tyrosine finally yields two types of thyroid hormone; T3 and T4.

This means that a deficiency of tyrosine can substantially reduce the production of thyroid hormone.[53] While our body is capable of producing a certain amount of tyrosine, it is better to supplement it by eating tyrosine-rich foods such as:

- Turkey
- Chicken
- Eggs
- Oats
- Nuts
- Beans

The Role of Vitamins

A great majority of people tend to think that iodine or selenium is the only nutrient required for making thyroid hormone. A lot of them are unaware that a mechanism exists in your thyroid gland that is responsible for actually drawing iodine into the thyroid gland. This mechanism can be compared to a doorway and is known as a symporter. For this symporter to work accurately, the presence of vitamin C and B2 is necessary. Failure of the symporter will not bring any iodine inside the thyroid and your body will suffer from hypothyroidism even if there is a surplus amount of iodine in the blood.

The role of vitamin D in thyroid health has been investigated in a study which concluded that lower levels of this vitamin can lead to a higher number of anti-thyroid antibodies. This suggests strong ties between vitamin D deficiency and the patients of Hashimoto's thyroiditis who generate this antibody. Both vitamin D and vitamin A are also important since they are required by T3 hormone to activate your body cells and increase the energy.

Given the importance of vitamins in an optimal thyroid functioning, it is crucial that you include lots of fruits and vegetables in your daily diet such as:

- Carrots
- Apricots
- Cantaloupe
- Sweet potatoes
- Kale, spinach, and leafy greens
- Winter squash
- Citrus fruits

The Role of Balanced Free Fatty Acids

The term "balanced free fatty acids" means taking omega-3 and omega-6 fatty acids in a balanced ratio. All the fatty acids are essential for a good health. However, the problem lies in the fact that most of the people particularly consume higher levels of omega-6 fatty acids by consuming processed foods.

This being said, the same people do not consume sufficient levels of omega- 3 fatty acids. This causes a disturbance in the ratio of these fatty acids which may affect the thyroid hormone synthesis. The optimal ratio of omega-6 to omega-3 fatty acids has to be 1:1 to 4:1, but because most people do not take care of this, the ratio often turns out to be 10:1 or sometimes 20:1. If you keep on consuming these fatty acids without any check and balance, it may lead to systemic inflammation and autoimmunity both of which form the basis of autoimmune thyroiditis.[54]

So, keep a check on the consumption of processed foods. At the same time, increase your omega-3 fatty acid intake by eating:

- Salmon
- Walnuts
- Canola oil
- Flaxseeds

- Chia seeds

Dietary goitrogens

Goitrogens refer to certain substances that interrupt the thyroid hormone production. These mainly include drugs and chemicals, however, goitrogens also exist naturally in some foods. Cruciferous vegetables such as cabbage and broccoli are said to have the highest concentration of goitrogens. As goitrogens are capable of aggravating the thyroid, eating these vegetables will most certainly exacerbate an underactive thyroid. However, this is possible only if the cause of hypothyroidism is iodine deficiency or if you consume ridiculously high amounts of goitrogens.

Assuming that you do not consume the dangerously high amount of cruciferous vegetables every day, there is no potential harm. In fact, these vegetables are packed with nutrients that will boost your health. Taking them frequently when you are already iodine-deficient may, however, bear consequences. Even if you have poor levels of iodine and still wish to consume cruciferous vegetables, you always have the option to cook them as cooking can drastically reduce the goitrogens levels. This has been proven by a small study in which the participants consumed 150 g of cooked Brussels sprouts every day for a month and experienced no side effects on the thyroid. [55,56]

Another concern regarding goitrogens is that they can stop the absorption of thyroid hormones if consumed simultaneously. Even if this is true, it is always better to take thyroid hormone on an empty stomach or at least one hour before having a meal. In this way, you can reduce your exposure to these so-called anti-thyroid agents.

Thyroid Supplements

Should you invest in some kind of thyroid supplements? This is a question that almost every thyroid patient asks, and rightly so because there is never an unbiased answer coming from a supplement manufacturer. To answer this question accurately, you need to examine 4 different nutritional aspects that these supplements may address; zinc, selenium, iodine, and vitamin B12.

1. Iodine Supplements

Contrary to the popular belief, iodine supplements are not necessary. Iodine deficiency alone is rarely the cause of hypothyroidism, especially in developed areas. The only exceptions to this are the women who are either pregnant or lactating. This is because the iodine requirements for such mothers increase by 60 percent. Females who find themselves in this category must definitely get help from iodine supplements as per the recommendations issued by the WHO. [57]

It is also important to bring to your notice that iodine supplements an sometimes irritate your thyroid, especially in the patients of Hashimoto's thyroiditis. Therefore, it is always wise to discuss with your doctor whether you should be taking iodine supplements or not.

2. Selenium Supplements

Selenium supplements are quite popular among the thyroid patients and can be of great help theoretically, especially if you suffer from a selenium deficiency. A literature review held in 2013 indicated a lack of evidence to encourage or discourage the use of these supplements for thyroid. Even though some studies did prove their usefulness, they were later found to be biased. [58]

In simpler words, the use of selenium supplements for thyroid health still requires research. This supplementation is promising for the patients with Graves' disease, but you need to try it for yourself to be more certain. It is also important to know that selenium supplements come with certain side effects such as fatigue, digestive issues, irritability, and hair loss, especially if used for a longer duration of time. 100 to 200 micrograms of selenium supplements is recommended for daily intake.

3. Zinc Supplements

A few studies have been performed regarding the usefulness of zinc supplementation on thyroid. These supplements have only been found useful in people suffering from goiter. But again, no solid recommendation can be given regarding its use or disuse. [59] 30 milligrams of zinc supplement is recommended to be used every day for hypothyroidism.

4. Vitamin B12 Supplements

Vitamin B12 is a micronutrient that can help in regulation of energy release. Low levels of this vitamin can make you lazy and lethargic so, theoretically speaking, vitamin B12 supplements can fight fatigue associated with hypothyroidism.

However, just like iodine, vitamin B12 deficiency is rarely a cause of hypothyroidism, especially in developed areas where people consume a wholesome diet on a daily basis. [60]

Your daily intake of vitamin B12 must be around 2.4 micrograms every day.

The Autoimmune Protocol Diet

The autoimmune protocol diet is a way treatment option for those suffering from Hashimoto's thyroiditis. This diet plan emphasizes on healing the gut by the elimination of certain foods that induce inflammation. It is particularly indicated in all autoimmune disorders. The autoimmune protocol diet is similar to Paleo diet in a way that it restricts the same kind of food.

So, how can you follow an autoimmune protocol diet?

What to Exclude

All types of every food item listed below needs to be avoided for a minimum of thirty days:

1. Eggs
2. Alcohol
3. Dairy
4. Legumes, seeds, and nuts
5. Grains
6. Every nightshade vegetable
7. Modern vegetable oils
8. Food additives
9. Products with artificial sweeteners or added sugar
10. NSAIDs such as aspirin

What to Include

The following list of foods can be taken as a part of the autoimmune protocol diet:

11. All vegetables except nightshades

12. Seafood rich in omega-3 fatty acids
13. High-quality meat
14. Fermented foods such as kefir or kimchi
15. High-quality fats including avocado, extra-virgin olive oil, etc
16. Small quantities of fruit

Lifestyle Changes for Hypothyroidism

Manage Stress

Psychological stress is undervalued when it comes to lifestyle management. Certain retrospective studies have indicated that up to 80 percent of the patients suffer from an emotional stress before acquiring a disease.[61] The logic behind this fact is that chronic stress can imbalance the hormones and alter the immune system.

Sleep Well

In addition to a sedentary lifestyle and poor diet, lack of sleep is also an important risk factor for many health problems. Prioritize your sleep if you wish to get rid of any health issue including hypothyroidism. Remember that your body needs a break and sleep is the best way to do it.

Eat Small Portions

To help eat smaller portions, try using smaller plates and spoons. Studies have proven that using small-sized plates and cutlery can reduce the amount of calories we consume.[62] This phenomenon has been termed as the Delbouef illusion and holds importance for those who wish to lose weight.

Stay Hydrated

Always keep a bottle of water with you whenever you leave the house. The more water you drink before meals, the lesser calories you consume overall. [63]

Practice Mindful Eating

Mindful eating involves being aware of every little physical cue and past experience regarding food. The foundation of mindful eating rests on a type of meditation known as mindfulness which encourages a person to consume lesser calories to maintain health.

Avoid Environmental Toxins

A lot of environmental toxins are structurally similar to thyroid hormones. Moreover, the thyroid gland has a natural tendency to attract metals and halogens such as iodine and selenium to produce thyroid hormone. While this process is important for hormone production, it may also lead to accumulation of harmful toxins that can damage the thyroid. So, try your best to steer clear of environmental toxins present in pesticides, plastics, heavy metals such as lead and mercury, and certain anti-bacterial agents like Triclosan.[64, 65, 66]

5. Hyperthyroidism: I'm a Ferrari!

The word hyper can be explained in a lot of ways. It refers to excessive, keyed up, or too much of a certain thing. All these words exactly depict the effect hyperthyroidism has on your body. In simple words, hyperthyroidism is a condition in which you feel constantly tensed, irritable and ready to explode any minute.[67] You will experience a condition as if you have just had eight cups of coffee and are always jazzed up.

This feeling is due to an overproduction of thyroid hormone in the body. Just like hypothyroidism reduces the production of thyroid hormone, a hyperactive thyroid produces too much of it. This leads to an overactive metabolism which fails to respond to decreased TSH levels.

Hyperthyroidism is not as common as hypothyroidism but both of these conditions are more likely to be seen in women as compared to men. The risk of hyperthyroidism increases as you age with the only exception of Graves' disease which strikes females of reproductive age, particularly between the age of twenty-five to fifty.[68]

Just like hypothyroidism, the signs and symptoms of hyperthyroidism cannot be detected easily, especially in older people. It presents itself in the most subtle way in this particular age group and makes it look like a completely different disease such as bowel issues or heart disease.

Hyperthyroidism requires urgent diagnosis and treatment because if left untreated, it can cause serious consequences. It can increase the risk of osteoporosis and heart diseases because an excessive amount of thyroid hormone can weaken your heart. Most of the people who experience the classic symptoms of hyperthyroidism are prescribed drugs to slow down the production of thyroid hormone. These drugs include radioactive iodine that destroys the abnormal part of the thyroid gland.[69] Sometimes, a surgery is also recommended before hyperthyroidism leads to any life-threatening complications.

Recognizing the Signs and Symptoms of Hyperthyroidism

The symptoms of hyperthyroidism appear gradually and may vary from one person to another. Most of the symptoms of an overactive thyroid such as an increased appetite or excessive thirst are not sufficient to suspect hyperthyroidism. Most of the time, people do not go to a doctor until they suffer signs such as shortness of breath or heart palpitations.

The following section addresses the signs and symptoms of hyperthyroidism experienced by most of the patients.[70,71]

Thyroid Enlargement

A hyperactive thyroid produces more and more hormone causing it to enlarge. This consequently leads to goiter which can be felt in the throat as a lump.

Heat Intolerance

Since too much thyroid hormone can increase the metabolism in your body. As the metabolic processes increase, more heat is produced. So, it may not be weird if you suddenly feel like opening the window when others are feeling chilly, or if you start wearing short sleeves instead of a woolen sweater.

Exhaustion

Your body is clearly overdriven due to hyperthyroidism which causes every system to exhaust eventually. This leads to shortness of breath as you climb the stairs or simply cross a street.

Emotional Alteration

An overactive hyperthyroid can not only make you physically exhausted but can also lead to certain emotional changes like depression, anxiety, irritability, and insomnia.

Changes in Perspiration

As the temperature in your body rises, the sweat glands become active. This causes increased perspiration and a consequent rise in thirst as your body attempts to compensate the fluid loss.

Constant Hunger

In hyperthyroidism, your body is using up energy at a speed higher than usual, making you cry out for more. This causes your appetite to increase and it will not be surprising if you catch yourself eating a lot more than usual.

Sudden Weight Loss

Even though a hyperactive thyroid increases your energy demand and forces you to eat more, you may find yourself losing weight. In case you are suffering from a severe form of Graves's disease, the weight loss can be extreme.

Tachycardia

Hyperthyroidism can alter your heart rhythms. Because this condition leads to overactivation of all the body systems, the heart also starts pumping a lot faster. This condition, known as tachycardia, is more prominent when you are working out or in a completely relaxed state.

Increased Heart Rate

If you have a habit of checking your pulse, you will observe that it has increased significantly. For example, if your pulse rate used to be 60 to 70 beats per minute in normal conditions, you may find it increased up to a 100 beats per minute in hyperthyroidism.

Hand Tremors

You may suddenly notice your hands shaking a lot more. It can be subtle or so severe that you are unable to hold a glass of water and drink it without spilling. These tremors are due to the overstimulation of nerves in your brain.

Muscle Weakness

Having too much thyroid hormone can break down the muscles causing extreme weakness. This feeling is particularly high in your limbs. If you have been a physically active person, hyperthyroidism may bring about some serious changes in your athletic capabilities.

Diarrhea

An overactive thyroid means overstimulation of all the body systems including the gastrointestinal (GI) tract. The mobility of the GI tract increases significantly causing the food to pass through it at an extremely high speed. This does not allow proper digestion of food or formation of feces. Resultantly, you suffer from diarrhea due to loose bowel movements.

Ophthalmic Problems

If you are suffering from Graves' disease, in particular, you are likely to suffer from certain eye problems. These problems predominantly comprise of eyelid retraction making your eyes bulge out. The eyes may also become puffy and are often watery. Sometimes, hyperthyroidism may even cause diplopia or double vision.

Menstrual Changes

If you are a female of childbearing age, hyperthyroidism may cause your periods to get lighter. You may even start skipping periods which can affect your ovulation and fertility as well.

Decreased Libido

In men, hyperthyroidism can alter your regular sperm cycle and induce infertility. The libido gets decreased when hyperthyroidism starts affecting testosterone levels in the body. Sometimes, it may cause gynecomastia or enlarged breasts in males due to a higher concentration of estrogen in the blood.

Skin Hives

Sometimes, an overactive thyroid may cause an itchy rash to appear anywhere on the skin. However, this is not something to worry about as it can be relieved with antihistamines.

Diagnosing Hyperthyroidism

Just like hypothyroidism, an overactive thyroid can only be detected with the help of a blood test. A TSH test is particularly recommended as it has a high sensitivity.[72] The symptoms of hyperthyroidism can easily be missed because they are often vague. However, if you start experiencing the classic signs of this problem- anxiety, a racing heart, shortness of breath- do not hesitate to book an appointment with your physician.

Your doctor might not check thyroid functions during a regular checkup so, it is entirely up to you to look for the symptoms and have knowledge about the risk factors that you are exposed to.
Hyperthyroidism can be diagnosed by your primary health care doctor but you may need a referral to an endocrinologist or sometimes, a thyroidiologist for better counsel.

The doctor will inquire you about the symptoms and examine the neck area to check if there is any goiter. An eye examination is also necessary to confirm the diagnosis of Graves' disease. The doctor will also look out for other physical manifestations of hyperthyroidism and ask a few questions about your family history or the history of any autoimmune problem.

If your blood TSH test shows abnormal results, this indicates that the pituitary gland in your body is constantly signaling the thyroid to slow down the production of thyroid hormone. In such a case, you will be asked to opt for a T4 test that determine the levels of freely circulating T4 in blood. If these levels are elevated, it means that there is too much thyroid hormone in your blood i.e. your thyroid is hyperactive. A blood test for estimating T3 levels can also be used in addition to a test for checking the presence of antibodies in case the doctor suspects you to have Graves' disease.

For diagnosing hyperthyroidism, it is also common to undergo certain tests that utilize radioactive iodine in small amounts. This is referred to as the radioactive iodine uptake (RAIU) test and is used to measure the rate at which the thyroid gland absorbs this iodine.[73] This is followed by a radioactive thyroid scan that determines if there is a structural problem with your thyroid such as the presence of a nodule. Such a scan can help determine if the nodule is of "hot" type which means that it is producing thyroid hormone and causing hyperthyroidism.

Medical Treatment of Hyperthyroidism

The goal of treatment in case of hyperthyroidism is to stop the thyroid overstimulation and there are a number of ways to achieve this. Radioactive iodine is one of the ways to destroy the malfunctioning part of the thyroid. Medicines can also be used to reduce the ability of your thyroid to generate hormones.

Lastly, a surgical method is opted in certain cases to remove some part of the thyroid gland.

If your primary health care doctor has diagnosed hyperthyroidism, you are likely to get referred to an endocrinologist. In contrast to hypothyroidism which can be treated by your basic health physician, managing hyperthyroidism requires a specialist as things can get a bit tricky. The specialist is responsible for outlining different therapeutic treatments for you.

The final decision of the treatment depends on several factors such as your age, the causative agent, the severity of disease, and the past medical history. It is important to understand the pros and cons of a certain therapy before choosing it. You may also seek an alternative option if you do not feel comfortable with the therapy recommended by your doctor. The following therapies may be used to treat hyperthyroidism:

Beta-blockers

Irrespective of what treatment fits you the best, your doctor may start the therapy by prescribing beta-adrenergic blocking agents to you. These medicines will not only cure an overactive thyroid but will also address the consequent symptoms. Beta-blockers are usually prescribed to treat problems like angina, hypertension, and coronary artery diseases. However, these agents are equally effective in treating hyperthyroidism since they can reduce the effect of thyroid hormone on your body tissues and may even provide relief in a couple of hours. While you explore your options to settle for a more permanent cure, beta-blockers can help you to relax. They will slow down the heart rate, reduce tremors, and decrease heart palpitations.

Propranolol was one of the earliest beta-blockers to come into the market but your doctor may choose from ten other varieties of this drug class that have been discovered so far.[74] Some types of beta-blockers that have been introduced to the market recently require one or two doses a day and can stay in your system for a much longer duration. On the other hand, some varieties of propranolol may require four doses per day to work.

Even though beta-blockers are safe, they too have certain side effects. Their long-term use can weaken your heart and cause excessive fatigue leading to exercise intolerance. If you are a patient of diabetes, beta-blockers may mask the symptoms of a low blood sugar. At the same time, they can make an episode of asthma a lot worse than it usually is. If you are on beta-blockers and suffer from symptoms such as wheezing, shortness of breath, vomiting, chest pain, or difficulty in breathing, contact your doctor immediately. Remember that beta-blockers are not suitable for long-term use in women who are pregnant or breastfeeding.

Radioactive Iodine Therapy

Administering radioactive iodine, a process known as radioactive ablation is a safe way to manage hyperthyroidism. It is a popular therapy in which a significant part of your thyroid is destroyed with the help of radioactive iodine, which thereby reduces the generation of thyroid hormone. The goal of this treatment is to make a patient euthyroid; a medical term that describes a thyroid gland producing the appropriate amount of hormone required by the body.[75] However, most of the times, the procedure ends up causing hypothyroidism, making you dependent on thyroid hormone for the rest of your life. In the long run, this is beneficial since it balances your hormones and makes you feel well.

The doctor is required to estimate the exact amount of radioactive iodine to cure hyperthyroidism in each individual patient. Even if this exact amount is used, the thyroid gland is likely to become overactive once again so most of the times, the doctors err towards the aggressive side. On the other hand, if the dose falls short, you are still likely to be hyperthyroid and would require another round to complete the treatment.

The procedure of using radioactive iodine is simple. You have to take a capsule containing radioactive iodine I-131, a potent isotope of iodine which can kill the overstimulated thyroid cells. The dosage of radioactive iodine is measured in units known as curies where one curie is equal to a thousand millicuries. Sometimes, another unit called becquerels is used for measuring the total amount of radioactive iodine to use. Normally, a dose of 185 to 1100 megabecquerels or 5 to 30 millicuries is enough to treat hyperthyroidism. A larger dose i.e. 30 to 75 millicuries may be warranted to manage a larger thyroid gland that is interfering with normal breathing. However, surgery is the preferred way of treatment if you suffer from a compressive goiter which may pounce upon the associated structures like trachea, esophagus, and the larger veins present in the neck. Larger doses are also recommended in cases where a surgery cannot be performed either because it is risky or the patient has not consented to it.

Anti-thyroid Drugs

Anti-thyroid drugs are the agents which can reduce the ability of a thyroid gland to form hormones. In this way, it can reduce the concentration of thyroid hormone in the blood and treat hyperthyroidism. Anti-thyroid drugs might be your only therapy in case of Graves' disease. In this disease, removal of the thyroid gland is not required because it is not large enough to compress the surrounding structures of the neck. Moreover, there are no troubling nodules that need to be removed in most of the cases. Under such circumstances, the anti-thyroid drugs allow an overactive thyroid to undergo spontaneous remission. However, the majority of patients for radioactive iodine therapy that has a better treatment outcome.

The benefits of using anti-thyroid drugs include a long-term remission of the thyroid gland without potentially damaging it. The disadvantage is that the doctor cannot ascertain the exact amoung of time required for these drugs to cause remission. Another side effect of using them includes side effects which can be fairly prominent in some patients. Using anti-thyroid drugs for a year or two can cause remission of the thyroid in up to 30 percent of the patients suffering from Graves's disease. Those who do not experience remission have a risk of relapsing. If you are not succeeding in overcoming hyperthyroidism, the doctor may switch you from anti-thyroid drugs to the radioactive iodine therapy that has lesser risks and a higher efficacy.

There are two main types of anti-thyroid drugs that are commonly used by the medical professionals; propylthiouracil (PTU) and methimazole (Tapazole).[76] Once you start taking any of these two drugs, it might take up to three months to start feeling a difference in the severity of symptoms.

Both PTU and methimazole have different mechanisms of action so, the doctor may prescribe the appropriate one depending upon your individual circumstances and health. For example, if you are pregnant, PTU is the drug of choice for hyperthyroidism because it has a lesser tendency to enter the fetal bloodstream and cause birth defects such as choanal atresia; a nasopharyngeal abnormality, and aplasia cutis; a rare scalp abnormality. Both of these abnormalities have been commonly linked to the use of methimazole in pregnant ladies.

Sometimes, the physicians prefer PTU as the drug of choice in patients with hyperthyroidism because it stops the peripheral conversion of T4 to a more active hormone T3. The recommended dose for PTU is 300 to 400 mg per day which is usually broken down into several doses because its duration of potency lasts up to eight hours only. Methimazole, on the other hand, is usually taken in a dose of 30 to 40 mg per day, all at one because its duration of action is much longer as compared to PTU. Moreover, methimazole might be related to some serious side effects but is less likely to cause it.

In some patients, anti-thyroid drugs may initiate allergic reactions such as joint pain, itching, and rashes. One out of every five hundred patients of hyperthyroidism taking anti-thyroid drug suffers from a reduction in the number of white blood cells. This condition can lower the body resistance to a great extent making the patient susceptible to a lot of other problems. It may even progress to a more severe condition known as agranulocytosis in which the white blood cells completely disappear from the blood.

Just to be sure that your white blood cell count is within normal ranges, the doctor will ask you to stop taking the medications and get tested if you acquire any signs of an infection such as a sore throat or a fever. If the anti-thyroid drugs are found to be lowering your white blood cell count, you will be asked to stop taking it immediately.

Another side of anti-thyroid drugs is liver damage, though this happens quite rarely. If you notice any symptoms of liver damage such as darkening of urine, yellowing of eyes, severe pain in the abdomen, or fatigue, stop taking the medication and contact the doctor immediately.

Natural Treatment of Hyperthyroidism

If the above-mentioned medical conditions tend to scare you off, opt for natural ways. Dietary restriction may not be able to treat hyperthyroidism naturally but it can definitely help speed up the process. The natural treatment for hyperthyroidism can be divided into two parts; things to limit and things to include in your daily diet.

Which Foods to Cut Off

There are certain dietary agents that contribute to the worsening of the thyroid. Some of these agents are explained below and need to be cut down in order to improve the health of your thyroid.

Iodine Food Sources

Iodine is mineral that your thyroid requires to produce hormones. As discussed before, the deficiency of iodine can lead to hypothyroidism. So, it is pretty clear that an excess of the same mineral can lead to hyperthyroidism too. This has also been documented in several case studies. A study recorded the case of a woman who drank kelp tea in large amounts every day for a month. This caused her iodine intake to increase between 3.8 to 6.6 times higher than the recommended allowance of 150 μg. It was not long before she developed multinodular goiter, a condition due to hyperthyroidism, and required urgent hospitalization. [77]

Another case-study discusses a woman who acquired hyperthyroidism soon after consuming a high-kelp diet. She had no previous medical history of thyroid issues which suggested that a high-iodine diet was the contributory cause. [78] Remember that iodine-rich foods can only lead to hyperthyroidism when eaten in larger amounts for a long period of time. Kelp, kelp tea, and supplemental iodine are dangerous for your thyroid so, speak with your doctor before using them.

Even if your doctor has scheduled you for a radioactive iodine therapy to get rid of hyperthyroidism, you will be instructed to restrict the intake of iodine. Iodine is commonly used in the feeding of animals. It is also used in food processing as a stabilizer. So, it may be a part of a lot of food items but in varying amounts. The highest sources of iodine are grains, certain types of bread, iodized salt, shellfish, pudding mixes, poultry, beef, and milk products.

Because a lot of food items that you consume every day happen to have iodine in them, it can be quite difficult to limit its use. To avoid such problems, following a low-iodine diet is recommended. Following is a food guide of what to eat for breakfast, lunch, dinner, and snacks if you wish to follow a low-iodine diet.

Breakfast

- Egg beaters
- Tea or black coffee
- Oatmeal with topping of honey, cinnamon, maple syrup, fruit, or walnuts
- Fruit/ fruit juices
- A slice toast

Lunch

- Matzo crackers
- Fruit or vegetable salads with vinegar/oil dressing

- Vegetable/chicken with rice soup
- Brown/white rice with vegetables
- Fruits; frozen, fresh, or canned
- Tea or black coffee

Dinner

- Baked or boiled potatoes
- Fruit or vegetable salad with vinegar/oil dressing
- Fruits
- 6 oz of roasted lamb, beef, veal, turkey, or pork
- Tea or black coffee

Snacks

- Dried fruits for example raisins
- Applesauce
- Fresh fruits/fruit juice
- Unsalted nuts
- Fresh vegetables (raw)

- Unsalted peanut butter (use it with crackers, carrot sticks, apple slices, or rice cakes)
- Unsalted crackers
- Bread and muffins baked at home

Gluten Food Sources

Before you know about how to follow a gluten-free diet, it is important to realize that there is a strong link between Graves' disease and Celiac disease. Many studies have proven that people with Celiac disease are much more prone to developing hyperthyroidism, Graves' disease to be more particular. [79] This connection stems from the link between intestinal inflammation, gluten and the initiation of autoimmune disease through molecular mimicry and inflammation. Some patients of hyperthyroidism may have a "silent" Celiac disease which means that they would not be exhibiting any intestinal symptoms related to this disease. This is particularly important if you are a patient and are hoping that your doctor knows this information and actually uses it during hyperthyroidism treatment.

Two cases studies have been documented individually in which two hyperthyroid patients were not responding to the standard therapeutic treatment for Graves' disease. In both cases, the patients were later diagnosed with the positive Celiac disease. [80, 81] What's more interesting is that they began responding to the same medications as soon as they went gluten-free. Other studies have also shown that a patient of Graves' disease has a 4.5 times higher risk of developing Celiac disease as compared to a healthy person.[82, 83].

Most of the time, the signs of Celiac disease are extra intestinal; they cannot be located within the GI tract but are more obvious anywhere else in the body. But why is it so important to find and treat Celiac disease in hyperthyroid patients? Treating

Celiac disease and removing gluten from the diet of a hyperthyroid patient can be extremely beneficial. This can increase the absorption of nutrients in the body and replenish any deficiencies that may be causing hyperthyroidism. It can also increase the absorption of medications and reduce inflammation in the body. Certain studies have even shown that going gluten-free may even reduce the anti-thyroid antibodies that may be causing Graves' disease in a vast majority of people.[84]

Now that the importance of a gluten-free diet in hyperthyroid patients have been established, the next important question to ask is for how long does this diet need to be followed?

This is where a lot of controversies arise. Most of the doctors recommend following a gluten-free diet for four to six weeks. Consider this a trial basis to check how much time your body would take to show improvements. For most of the people, restricting gluten for six weeks is sufficient to subside most of the symptoms but there are some problems with it. The first problem is that you must not be relying on the symptoms alone. Gluten might be damaging to your intestinal lining but it does not lead to any overt symptoms, so it is likely that you may not feel any improvements as you switch to a gluten-free diet. Additionally, if gluten is producing problems such as a leaky gut in your body, you may need to continue avoiding it up to six months or even longer.

What can you eat during a gluten-free dietary protocol? Some natural gluten-free foods that you may consume are:

- Fruits and vegetables
- Eggs
- Nuts, seeds, and beans (unprocessed)
- Unprocessed lean meats
- Low-fat dairy products

You may eat grains and starches too, but with the following exceptions:

- Rye
- Barley
- Wheat
- Oats
- Triticale

When you are purchasing processed foods, always read the labels to check if they have gluten. Foods that contain the 5 types of grain mentioned above or any ingredient that has been derived from them must be avoided. Look for food items that have been labeled as gluten-free by the Food and Drug Administration as they have less than 20 parts per million of gluten in them.

Soy and Goitrogens

Goitrogens refer to substances that can inhibit your thyroid gland and soy is one of them.[85] Soy can interfere with the normal functioning of the thyroid by stopping thyroid peroxidase (TPO) enzyme. This enzyme is required by the thyroid gland to iodinate tyrosine to synthesize thyroid hormones. Soy, by the virtue of the two isoflavones- genistein and daidzein- can block this enzyme and the consequent hormonal synthesis. As the thyroid hormones stop being produced, the thyroid glands begin to enlarge, ultimately leading to goiter.

According to the Food and Agriculture Organization of the United Nations, soy is included in the top 8 food allergens. Up till now, almost 16 potential protein allergens have been identified in the composition of soy.[86] It is said that only 50 percent of the children who are allergic to soy manage to outgrow their allergy which means that the rest of them continue to have it in the later stages of life. Moreover, a lot of people who do not have an IgE-mediated allergy to soy may exhibit a different pathway, preferably an IgG-mediated one.

What exactly happens if you are a hyperthyroid patient with a potential soy allergy and you keep consuming it nevertheless? The problem with eating a particular food item that you are allergic to will result in inflammation and inflammation can, in turn, interfere in the process of healing. Even if you try to run a food allergy test, these tests do not always provide accurate results. So, it is better for you to avoid soy altogether.

Another reason why you should be avoiding soy is that it contains phytates. Phytic acid refers to an anti-nutrient that is commonly found in legumes, seeds, and grains. Studies have indicated that phytates present in soy can decrease the absorption of calcium and iron in the body and the deficiencies may lead to a malfunctioning thyroid.

Other foods that may be considered as goitrogens include plants belonging to the genus Brassica such a watercress, kale, cabbage, Brussels sprouts, turnips, broccoli, and cauliflowers. These vegetables are more harmful to the patients of hypothyroidism, however, every case has to be analyzed individually. Because Brassica vegetables can block the iodine uptake, this can have a negative effect on the thyroid gland of a person suffering from Graves' disease. These plants are commonly goitrogenic when consumed in raw forms and must always be cooked before consumption. The usage must be based on the analysis of every case individually.

The consumption of goitrogens must be minimized if you suffer from hyperthyroidism. However, in some cases, it is better to completely avoid them. This is true for certain goitrogenic foods which are worse than others. For example, cruciferous vegetables are generally healthy for your body despite the fact that they are goitrogenic. Consuming them on an occasional basis and in cooked form is okay for your body. On the other hand, soy is something that needs to be avoided completely as eating it in high amounts can cause certain health problems.

Which Foods to Include in Diet

Now that you are clear about which foods to avoid during hyperthyroidism management, it is time to discuss the food options that are must to include in your diet if you are considering to opt for a natural thyroid management.

Magnesium Food Sources

Why do you need more magnesium in hyperthyroidism? Magnesium is an important cofactor for calcitonin; a hormone generated by the parafollicular cells of the thyroid. Some studies have shown that an excessive level of thyroid hormone in the blood i.e. hyperthyroidism can reduce the absorption of magnesium in the blood. This means that people who suffer from hyperthyroidism are likely to be deficient in this mineral. This is why a lot of people suffering from Grave' disease observe a huge difference in the heart palpitations when they are supplemented with magnesium.

The recommended daily intake of magnesium is around 400 mg but this is on the low side, just as in case of every other mineral and vitamin. The actual intake of magnesium must be around 600t to 800 mg which you can get from natural foods. However, if a doctor suggests a possible magnesium deficiency for you, you may be required to take supplements.

Some good food sources of magnesium that can be included in the daily diet are:

- Quinoa
- Peanuts
- Black beans
- Almonds
- Edamame
- Cashews
- Leafy greens such as spinach
- Whole wheat and other whole grains

Calcium Food Sources

Research has demonstrated that an abnormal thyroid function has an ability to alter the metabolism of calcium. Back in 1929, it was also proposed that the excretion of calcium via urine or feces increases to a great extent in the patients with hyperthyroidism. This proposition is now supported by the recent scientific evidence as well.

Losing calcium from the body puts a patient of hyperthyroidism at an increased risk of acquiring osteoporosis. This is because an uncontrolled hyperthyroidism can lead to a decreased bone mineral density, pull out both calcium and phosphorus from the bones and excrete a large amount of calcium out of the body. Because your bones require phosphorus and calcium to maintain their health, a deficiency of either of these nutrients can make bones less dense. So, while you are suffering from hyperthyroidism, your body is literally begging you for calcium. The following natural foods can provide you calcium while avoiding gluten:

- Vegetables with high calcium content such as kale, mustard, bok choy, cabbages, and turnip greens
- Gluten-free gains such as amaranth, teff, and cornmeal
- Canned fish such as salmon and sardines
- Almonds, sesame seeds, brazil nuts, and chia seeds
- Calcium-fortified almond milk and orange juice

With so many options to choose from, it will not be hard to get the recommended amount of calcium every day i.e. 1000 mg per day. However, if supplementation is necessary, it is advised to take supplements in quantities sufficient to fill the gap between what you are acquiring from diet and the recommended calcium intake. In most of the cases, this gap is around 250 mg or less every day but in case of hyperthyroidism, it might be a lot higher.

Vitamin D Food Sources

The deficiency of vitamin D has been associated with a lot of autoimmune diseases including Graves' disease. Vitamin D is responsible for balancing the Th1 and Th2 cells of the immune system. This is accomplished as vitamin D influences the T3 cells and thereby governs the differentiation and expression of both Th1 and Th2 cells.[87] Vitamin D deficiency is also related to autoimmune thyroid disease and benefits the autoimmune-mediated dysfunction of the thyroid.

Scientists have discovered that vitamin D can silence the inflammatory signals being generated in a human body. At the same time, it makes the immune system a lot more flexible. This means that the immune system is less likely to get imbalanced and cause autoimmunity. It has also been found that low levels of vitamin D increase the risk of anti-thyroid antibodies production in the body. Not to forget that these autoantibodies form the basis of

Graves' disease, a condition in which your thyroid becomes hyperactive.

Vitamin D is so important for your body that its deficiency can even interfere with other therapeutic interventions for hyperthyroidism. A study published in in the Journal of Endocrinological Investigation has suggested that the patients of Graves' disease having a vitamin D level below 20 ng/ml are more likely to suffer from a failure during the radioiodine therapy; one of the most effective interventions for hyperthyroidism.[88] This suggests that vitamin D is not only crucial for the proper working of thyroid but is also required for other hyperthyroidism treatments to work.

The normal range for vitamin D levels in the body is 30 to 100 ng/ml. However, new evidence suggests that that optimal level of vitamin D for stronger bones and healthy body is around 35 ng/ml. People suffering from autoimmune diseases such as

Graves' disease may require a dose higher than this. Replenishment of vitamin D levels for months may turn out to be quite helpful in the patients with hyperthyroidism. You must work with your doctor to decide the best blood level and vitamin D dosage for you, especially if you have a parathyroid problem or an underlying kidney disease simultaneously.

Some best food sources of vitamin D include:

- Oily fish for example sardines, salmon, herring, pilchards, kippers, trout, and eel
- Meat, egg yolk, offal, and milk
- Vitamin D fortified yogurt and margarine
- Cod liver oil
- Orange juice and almond milk
- Oysters and shrimps

Additionally, bask in the sunshine for 15 to 20 minutes every day to naturally boost the production of vitamin D in your body.

Lifestyle Changes for Hyperthyroidism

Avoid Smoking

Smoking puts you at the risk of acquiring a thyroid problem if you don't have it and increases the risk of developing thyroid-related eye disease if you already have hyperthyroidism. It can also increase your exposure to carcinogens and heavy metals which can worsen Graves' disease and make life more difficult. So, it is better to quit smoking in order to manage hyperthyroidism effectively.

Cut Down on Caffeine

It is quite obvious to remove caffeine from the diet if you suffer from an overactive thyroid. Anything with stimulating properties must be excluded or at the very least, significantly reduced from your body, at least till the time your thyroid gains balance again.

Limit Alcohol Consumption

If you suffer from hyperthyroidism or Graves' disease or even if you are at a risk of acquiring either, it is wise to reduce your alcohol consumption to one glass per week. If you occasionally indulge in more than one glass of alcohol per week, ensure that you drink a lot of water and beet juice before and after consuming alcohol. Also, be careful not to take aspirin after consuming alcohol to handle the hangover as it can deteriorate health.

Try Essential Oils

Essential oils possess extraordinary healing abilities and can help manage hyperthyroidism. The best essential oils to use are:

- Lemongrass
- Myrrh

- Sandalwood
- Wintergreen
- Frankincense
- Black Spruce

These oils can induce calmness, relaxation and inner vision and may also treat restlessness associated with hyperthyroidism. The best way to use these essential oils is with the help of a diffuser. You can also add them in olive oil, body butter, or beeswax and apply on the skin to balance your emotional state.

Exercise More

Exercise is a great way to mentally calm a patient with hyperthyroidism. Tai Chi, meditation, and yoga are wonderful options to opt for mental relaxation. These are all gentle forms of exercises and do not stress your body any more than it already is. In fact, these exercise programs make you more mindful of what you are doing and slow down the internal systems that have been greatly disturbed by hyperthyroidism/.

It is also recommended to include weight-bearing exercises in your daily schedule to strengthen bones and build muscles. This is because hyperthyroidism can reduce your calcium intake and may lead to muscle loss.

6. A Guide to Thyroid Tests

Thyroid tests typically involve three domains; blood tests, radioactive iodine tests, and thyroid imaging scans. Most of the tests aim at determining the thyroid functioning. Imaging tests are sometimes required to investigate structural problems such as a goiter.

Blood Tests

Functional thyroid disease, including hyperthyroidism and hypothyroidism, are characterized by imbalanced hormones. Therefore, blood tests are required to determine if the hypothalamic-pituitary-thyroid axis is working properly.

1. TSH (Thyroid-stimulating Hormone) Test

It is usually the first step to examine the thyroid-stimulating hormone (TSH), a hormone produced by the pituitary gland which regulates the amount of thyroid hormone produced. Recent advances have led to the development of a more sensitive TSH to check if you have a thyroid disorder. If this test comes out to be normal, it means that your TSH levels are normal. An abnormally high concentration, however, indicates that your pituitary gland is repeatedly sending signals to your failing thyroid gland and you are probably a patient of hypothyroidism. In contrast, low TSH levels indicate that your thyroid gland is overactive and secreting too much hormones.[89]

2. T4 (Thyroxine) Tests

T4, also known as thyroxine, is a thyroid hormone that exists in two forms. As the thyroid secretes it, it is present in "bound" form and is not available to your body cells. Only 1% of this hormone is "free" which means that it can be used by the body immediately. Since bound form constitutes almost 99% of the total T4 hormone, it constitutes the total amount of T4 circulating in the blood.

Free T4 (FT4) tests are, however, more important and performed along with TSH and provides an account of how your thyroid is working. For example, elevated levels of TSH with low FT4 indicate primary hypothyroidism which means that the problem lies in your thyroid gland. If the levels of TSH and FT4 are low, this means that the problem lies in your pituitary gland and you suffer from secondary hypothyroidism.[90]

Lastly, a low TSH and with high level of FT4 means that your T4 levels are extremely high. In such circumstances, a radioactive iodine test is recommended for specific diagnosis.

3. T3 (Triiodothyronine) Tests

Just like T4, most of the T3 present in your blood is in bound form. There are several tests to measure this hormone such as the total T3 test which measures the amount of circulating T3, or the Free T3 (FT3) test which investigates the total amount of free T3 hormone readily available to your body cells. In most of the cases, a combination of both tests is required. T3 tests are not generally used to establish a diagnosis of hypothyroidism because the T3 levels are usually the last to fall. However, they are sometimes used to diagnose hyperthyroidism and its severity.[91]

4. Thyroid Antibody Tests

Antibody tests are used to diagnose an autoimmune disorder of the thyroid gland. If the T4 and TSH levels suggest that you are hypothyroid, your physician may want to test you for the presence of anti-TPO or anti-Tg antibodies in the blood. Anti-Tg antibodies target thyroglobulin, an important component required for the production of thyroid hormones. Anti-TPO antibodies, on the other hand, target thyroid peroxidase; an enzyme that catalyzes the production of thyroid hormones. The presence of these antibodies suggest that you are suffering from Hashimoto's thyroiditis.

Conversely, if you have been diagnosed with hyperthyroidism, the doctor will want to check for any antibodies targeted against the TSH receptors present on the thyroid gland. If the antibodies are present, you may be diagnosed as a case of Graves' disease.[92]

5. TRH (Thyrotropin-releasing Hormone) Test

TRH or Thyrotropin-releasing hormone) is a hormone secreted by your hypothalamus that stimulates the TSH production by the pituitary gland. In most of the cases, a TRH test is not required but if your doctor is unable to locate the problem in thyroid or pituitary glands, it may be needed.[93] The test requires a blood sample for TSH in which TRH is administered intravenously. Because the TSH tests have become ultrasensitive these days, TRH tests are not used anymore.

Radioactive Iodine Tests

Radioactive iodine tests indicate the ability of thyroid gland to attract iodine from the blood and use it to produce hormones. These tests are used when your body contains too much thyroid hormone and are aimed at detecting nodules. You are provided with a small amount of radioactive iodine, mostly Iodine-131 that you consume orally. Once it gets into your system, the thyroid gland pulls it from blood routinely but in this case, the doctors are able to trace the whole process. This allows them to determine how well your thyroid gland is concentrating iodine.[94] Radioactive iodine tests are not needed in case of hypothyroidism as the blood tests are sufficient to find the cause.

Radioactive Thyroid Scan

This test is usually performed to check any structural abnormalities in the thyroid. It resembles the radioactive iodine tests in a lot of ways. You are provided with a small amount of radioactive iodine, either in the form of an injection or a capsule. In this test, however, a special camera is sued to obtain pictures of the thyroid gland from 3 separate angles. An abnormal thyroid scan may present as a large or a small thyroid gland. It can also spot the areas in the thyroid gland where there is abnormally high or low activity.

A thyroid scan is also performed to check if a nodule is active or whether it is a "hot" nodule i.e. it is producing thyroid hormone or a "cold" one which means that it is not producing any hormone on its own.

Specific Tests for Hypothyroidism

Vitamin D Levels

Blood tests are the only way of measuring the levels of vitamin D in your body. The lab test specifically recommended for this purpose is known as 25(OH)D blood test. You can get this test performed in three ways:

- Ask your doctor to perform it on you. While you are doing so, ask specifically for a 25(OH)D blood test because this is the only way to know if you are getting sufficient amount of this vitamin.

- Ask for an in-home test kit. All you need to do is prick your finger and place a drop of blood on blotting paper. This paper is sent to the laboratory for assessment of vitamin D.

- You can also order an online test via certain American websites, perform the test at home, and visit a nearby lab for results.

Minerals Levels

The best way for a hypothyroid patient to check their minerals levels is by a hair minerals analysis. A hair analysis utilizes a special technique to closely examine your hair with the help of a microscope. The result can speak volumes about your health and daily habits. There are a number of ways to perform this test and your doctor is the one to suggest the most suitable one according to your individual needs.

The importance of a hair analysis in the patients of hypothyroidism is that it can help evaluate any mineral deficiencies that may be causing the problem. For example, any disturbance in the calcium to potassium ratio can disturb the cellular response towards the thyroid hormone and this disturbance can be detected by hair analysis. In a similar way, this test can detect and depict the deficiency of any other mineral that may be causing an underactive thyroid.

Digestive Problems

For thyroid gland to work properly, your body must be capable of converting T4 into T3 hormone. About 20 percent of this process occurs inside your intestines under the assistance of the colonic bacteria. This means that any disturbance in the bacterial colonies can be a cause of your hypothyroidism. If you suffer from any type of digestive problem, there is a good possibility that it is harming your thyroid. Gas, bloating, constipation, and heartburn are some of the signs of an underlying digestive issue. However, for a more reliable result, you can perform a test at home.

You can check the digestive problems at home by a transit time test. Normally, it takes 18 to 24 hours for food to pass through the digestive system, and if it takes longer than this, there is some digestive problem. Purchase a product called "activated charcoal" which can turn your feces dark gray or black. Swallow four of its capsules and write down the exact time and date when you took them. Now, wait for your feces to turn black and note the difference between the two time periods. If this difference is lesser than 18 hours or greater than 24 hours, this means that there is a digestive problem to look out for.

A more professional way for detecting digestive issues is by getting a full stool analysis under the supervision of a medical doctor. This can tell you if there are any digestive infections that may be affecting the thyroid gland.

Adrenal Tests

Adrenal glands are referred to as the life-saving organs since they control the hormonal system of your body and help you manage stressful situations. They are responsible for the famous "fight or flight" response and help secrete different hormones including adrenaline, testosterone, and cortisol. Adrenal problems or adrenal fatigue can set off an autoimmune inflammatory response in the body which can harm all the body organs and can even make a thyroid problem a lot worse.

The best way to assess adrenal fatigue is through a cortisol test. In this test, the doctor performs an analysis of your urine, blood, or saliva to detect the cortisol levels. The test is repeated with four different samples to check the levels over the time span of 24 hours.

7. Shopping: An Add-to-Cart Kindda Day

If you are a thyroid patient and are about to take a trip to the supermarket, be sure to add these things to your groceries.

Fruit & Vegetables

Bananas

Berries (fresh/frozen)

Mango (fresh/frozen)

Pumpkin

Lemon/ lemon juice

Sweet potatoes

Apples

Baby spinach

Yellow/brown onions

Garlic

Carrots

Celery

Zucchinis

Bell peppers

Cucumber

Chipotle peppers

Alternatives to Dairy/Milk

Milk (skimmed or full cream)

Unsweetened almond milk

Feta cheese

Greek yogurt

Cottage cheese

Cheddar cheese

Animal Products

Eggs

Salmon fillet

Minced beef

Extra firm tofu

Lamb

Turkey

Chicken breast

Nuts & Seeds

Roasted almonds

Brazil nuts

Sesame seeds

Sunflower seeds

Unsalted cashews

Pasta, Rice & Grains

White/brown rice

Chia seeds

Quinoa

Fats and Oils

Butter

Balsamic vinegar

Extra virgin olive oil

Tinned/Bottled Foods

Black beans

Peanut butter

Soy sauce

Light/regular coconut milk (canned)

Diced tomatoes

Maple syrup

Canned tuna

Mayonnaise

Honey

Vegetable or chicken stock

Beans

Black beans

Azuki beans

Pinto beans

Mung beans

Condiments & Spices

Cinnamon

Cumin

Peppermint

Cocoa powder

Chilli powder

Cilantro

Vanilla extract

Paprika

Greek seasoning

8. Conclusion: Remembering What it is Like to Feel Normal

Living with a chronic thyroid issue can be difficult. Some days are surprisingly better while some are just impossible to get through. Will you be depressed, feel fatigued, gain weight or become frustrated? Yes, but by getting your thyroid medicines, eating well, taking your vitamins, and working out, it is possible to feel normal again. Even if you are still not feeling well, do not lose hope. Perhaps it is time to go for a different medication. There are several medicines for a thyroid problem. Remember that it is not a one-size-fits-all type of situation. It may be frustrating in the beginning, but you will soon figure it all out. You may find out that a gluten-free diet works for you. You may benefit from switching to Armor or trying a different T3 medication in your treatment regimen. You would not know it until you try. So, clean up your diet, get a good bedtime routine, indulge in self-care activities and take your medicines timely. Go to the doctor when it is necessary. Advocate for yourself. Take good care of yourself. You deserve to feel better!

References

1. Cavalieri RR. Iodine metabolism and thyroid physiology: current concepts. Thyroid. 1997 Apr; 7(2):177-81.
2. Monaco F. Classification of thyroid diseases: suggestions for a revision. The Journal of Clinical Endocrinology & Metabolism. 2003 Apr 1;88(4):1428-32.
3. Weetman AP. Graves' disease. New England Journal of Medicine. 2000 Oct 26;343(17):1236-48.
4. Winsa B, Adami HO, Bergstrom R, Gamstedt A, Dahlberg PA, Adamson U, Jansson R, Karlsson A. Stressful life events and Graves' disease. The Lancet. 1991 Dec 14;338(8781):1475-9.Smith B, Hall R. Thyroid-stimulating immunoglobulins in graves'disease. The Lancet. 1974 Aug 24;304(7878):427-30.
5. Smith B, Hall R. Thyroid-stimulating immunoglobulins in graves'disease. The Lancet. 1974 Aug 24;304(7878):427-30.
6. Stenszky V, Kozma L, Balazs CS, Rochlitz SZ, Bear JC, Farid NR. The genetics of Graves' disease: HLA and disease susceptibility. The Journal of Clinical Endocrinology & Metabolism. 1985 Oct 1;61(4):735-40.

7. Hanafusa T, Chiovato L, Doniach D, Pujol-Borrell R, Russell RC, Bottazzo gf. Aberrant expression of hla-dr antigen on thyrocytes in graves'disease: relevance for autoimmunity. The Lancet. 1983 Nov 12;322(8359):1111-5.
8. Thyroid Nodules and Swellings [Internet]. British Thyroid foundation. Available from: http://www.btf-thyroid.org/information/leaflets/32-thyroid-nodules-and-swellings-guide
9. Krohn K, Führer D, Bayer Y, Eszlinger M, Brauer V, Neumann S, Paschke R. Molecular pathogenesis of euthyroid and toxic multinodular goiter. Endocrine reviews. 2005 Jun;26(4):504-24.
10. Thyroid Nodules and Swellings [Internet]. British Thyroid foundation. Available from: http://www.btf-thyroid.org/information/leaflets/32-thyroid-nodules-and-swellings-guide
11. Monaco F. Classification of thyroid diseases: suggestions for a revision. The Journal of Clinical Endocrinology & Metabolism. 2003 Apr 1;88(4):1428-32.
12. Hershman JM. Overview of the Thyroid Gland [Internet]. Merck Manuals. Merck; Available from: https://www.merckmanuals.com/home/hormonal-and-metabolic-disorders/thyroid-gland-disorders/overview-of-the-thyroid-gland?qt=thyroxine&alt=sh

13. Tamai h, Suemastu h, Kurokawa n, Esaki m, Ikemi t, Matsuzuka f, Kuma k, Nagataki s. Alterations in circulating thyroid hormones and thyrotropin after complete thyroidectomy. The Journal of Clinical Endocrinology & Metabolism. 1979 Jan 1;48(1):54-8.
14. Hashimoto's Disease [Internet]. The National Institute of Diabetes and Digestive and Kidney Diseases. NIH; Available from: https://www.niddk.nih.gov/health-information/endocrine-diseases/hashimotos-disease
15. Hashimoto's Disease [Internet]. Women's Health. Office on Women's Health; Available from: https://www.womenshealth.gov/a-z-topics/hashimotos-disease
16. Monaco F. Classification of thyroid diseases: suggestions for a revision. The Journal of Clinical Endocrinology & Metabolism. 2003 Apr 1;88(4):1428-32.
17. Persani L. Central hypothyroidism: pathogenic, diagnostic, and therapeutic challenges. The Journal of Clinical Endocrinology & Metabolism. 2012 Sep 1;97(9):3068-78.
18. Donaldson M, Jones J. Optimising outcome in congenital hypothyroidism; current opinions on best practice in initial assessment and subsequent management. Journal of

clinical research in pediatric endocrinology. 2013 Mar;5(Suppl 1):13.
19. Persani L. Central hypothyroidism: pathogenic, diagnostic, and therapeutic challenges. The Journal of Clinical Endocrinology & Metabolism. 2012 Sep 1;97(9):3068-78.
20. Monaco F. Classification of thyroid diseases: suggestions for a revision. The Journal of Clinical Endocrinology & Metabolism. 2003 Apr 1;88(4):1428-32.
21. Garber JR, Cobin RH, Gharib H, Hennessey JV, Klein I, Mechanick JI, Pessah-Pollack R, Singer PA, Woeber for the American Association of Clinical Endocrinologists and American Thyroid Association Taskforce on Hypothyroidism in Adults KA. Clinical practice guidelines for hypothyroidism in adults: cosponsored by the American Association of Clinical Endocrinologists and the American Thyroid Association. Thyroid. 2012 Dec 1;22(12):1200-35.
22. Burrow GN, Burke WR, Himmelhoch JM, Spencer RP, Hershman JM. Effect of lithium on thyroid function. The Journal of Clinical Endocrinology & Metabolism. 1971 May 1;32(5):647-52.
23. Burman PI, TÖTTERMAN TH, Öberg K, Karlsson FA. Thyroid autoimmunity in patients on long term therapy with leukocyte-derived

interferon. The Journal of Clinical Endocrinology & Metabolism. 1986 Nov 1;63(5):1086-90.
24. Definition of thyroid [Internet]. SensAgent. SenAgent Corporation; Available from: http://dictionary.sensagent.com/THYROID/en-en/
25. Persani L. Central hypothyroidism: pathogenic, diagnostic, and therapeutic challenges. The Journal of Clinical Endocrinology & Metabolism. 2012 Sep 1;97(9):3068-78.
26. Hypothyroidism (Underactive Thyroid) [Internet]. The National Institute of Diabetes and Digestive and Kidney Diseases. NIH; Available from: https://www.niddk.nih.gov/health-information/endocrine-diseases/hypothyroidism
27. Garber JR, Cobin RH, Gharib H, Hennessey JV, Klein I, Mechanick JI, Pessah-Pollack R, Singer PA, Woeber for the American Association of Clinical Endocrinologists and American Thyroid Association Taskforce on Hypothyroidism in Adults KA. Clinical practice guidelines for hypothyroidism in adults: cosponsored by the American Association of Clinical Endocrinologists and the American Thyroid

Association. Thyroid. 2012 Dec 1;22(12):1200-35.
28. Joanna Klubo-Gwiezdzinska, Leonard Wartofsky. Medical Clinics of North America. Thyroid Emergencies. Volume 96, Issue 2. 2012 385-403.
29. Joanna Klubo-Gwiezdzinska, Leonard Wartofsky. Medical Clinics of North America. Thyroid Emergencies. Volume 96, Issue 2. 2012 385-403.
30. Garber JR, Cobin RH, Gharib H, Hennessey JV, Klein I, Mechanick JI, Pessah-Pollack R, Singer PA, Woeber for the American Association of Clinical Endocrinologists and American Thyroid Association Taskforce on Hypothyroidism in Adults KA. Clinical practice guidelines for hypothyroidism in adults: cosponsored by the American Association of Clinical Endocrinologists and the American Thyroid Association. Thyroid. 2012 Dec 1;22(12):1200-35.
31. So M, MacIsaac RJ, Grossmann M. Investigation and management.
32. Garber JR, Cobin RH, Gharib H, Hennessey JV, Klein I, Mechanick JI, Pessah-Pollack R, Singer PA, Woeber for the American Association of Clinical Endocrinologists and American Thyroid Association Taskforce on Hypothyroidism in Adults KA. Clinical practice guidelines for

hypothyroidism in adults: cosponsored by the American Association of Clinical Endocrinologists and the American Thyroid Association. Thyroid. 2012 Dec 1;22(12):1200-35.
33. So M, MacIsaac RJ, Grossmann M. Investigation and management.
34. https://www.mayoclinic.org/drugs-supplements/levothyroxine-oral-route/side-effects/drg-20072133
35. Ko YJ, Kim JY, Lee J, Song HJ, Kim JY, Choi NK, Park BJ. Levothyroxine dose and fracture risk according to the osteoporosis status in elderly women. Journal of Preventive Medicine and Public Health. 2014 Jan;47(1):36.
36. Siegmund W, Spieker K, Weike AI, Giessmann T, Modess C, Dabers T, Kirsch G, Sänger E, Engel G, Hamm AO, Nauck M. Replacement therapy with levothyroxine plus triiodothyronine (bioavailable molar ratio 14: 1) is not superior to thyroxine alone to improve well-being and cognitive performance in hypothyroidism. Clinical endocrinology. 2004 Jun 1;60(6):750-7.
37. Clyde PW, Harari AE, Getka EJ, Shakir KM. Combined levothyroxine plus liothyronine compared with levothyroxine alone in primary hypothyroidism: a randomized controlled trial. Jama. 2003 Dec 10;290(22):2952-8.

38. Walsh JP, Shiels L, Lim EM, Bhagat CI, Ward LC, Stuckey BG, Dhaliwal SS, Chew GT, Bhagat MC, Cussons AJ. Combined thyroxine/liothyronine treatment does not improve well-being, quality of life, or cognitive function compared to thyroxine alone: a randomized controlled trial in patients with primary hypothyroidism. The Journal of Clinical Endocrinology & Metabolism. 2003 Oct 1;88(10):4543-50.

39. FDA regulation of drugs versus dietary supplements [Internet]. American Cancer Society. Leo and Gloria Rosen family; Available from: https://www.cancer.org/treatment/treatments-and-side-effects/complementary-and-alternative-medicine/dietary-supplements/fda-regulations.html

40. Study: 'Thyroid Support' Supplements May Be Risky [Internet]. WebMd. WebMD LLC; Available from: https://www.webmd.com/women/news/20111028/study-thyroid-support-supplements-may-be-risky#1

41. Jonklaas J, Bianco AC, Bauer AJ, Burman KD, Cappola AR, Celi FS, Cooper DS, Kim BW, Peeters RP, Rosenthal MS, Sawka AM. Guidelines for the treatment of hypothyroidism: prepared by the american thyroid association task force on thyroid

hormone replacement. Thyroid. 2014 Dec 1;24(12):1670-751.
42. Bach-Huynh TG, Nayak B, Loh J, Soldin S, Jonklaas J. Timing of levothyroxine administration affects serum thyrotropin concentration. The Journal of Clinical Endocrinology & Metabolism. 2009 Oct 1;94(10):3905-12.
43. Bolk N, Visser TJ, Nijman J, Jongste IJ, Tijssen JG, Berghout A. Effects of evening vs morning levothyroxine intake: a randomized double-blind crossover trial. Archives of internal medicine. 2010 Dec 13;170(22):1996-2003.
44. Rajput R, Chatterjee S, Rajput M. Can levothyroxine be taken as evening dose? Comparative evaluation of morning versus evening dose of levothyroxine in treatment of hypothyroidism. Journal of thyroid research. 2011;2011.
45. Ala S, Akha O, Kashi Z, Asgari H, Bahar A, Sasanpour N. Dose administration time from before breakfast to before dinner affect thyroid hormone levels?. Caspian journal of internal medicine. 2015;6(3):134.
46. Guariso G, Conte S, Presotto F, Basso D, Brotto F, POZZA LV, Pedini B, Betterle C. Clinical, subclinical and potential autoimmune diseases in an Italian population of children with coeliac disease. Alimentary

pharmacology & therapeutics. 2007 Nov;26(10):1409-17.
47. Cosnes J, Cellier C, Viola S, Colombel JF, Michaud L, Sarles J, Hugot JP, Ginies JL, Dabadie A, Mouterde O, Allez M. Incidence of autoimmune diseases in celiac disease: protective effect of the gluten-free diet. Clinical Gastroenterology and Hepatology. 2008 Jul 1;6(7):753-8.
48. Caldwell KL, Miller GA, Wang RY, Jain RB, Jones RL. Iodine status of the US population, national health and nutrition examination survey 2003–2004. Thyroid. 2008 Nov 1;18(11):1207-14.
49. Cosnes J, Cellier C, Viola S, Colombel JF, Michaud L, Sarles J, Hugot JP, Ginies JL, Dabadie A, Mouterde O, Allez M. Incidence of autoimmune diseases in celiac disease: protective effect of the gluten-free diet. Clinical Gastroenterology and Hepatology. 2008 Jul 1;6(7):753-8.
50. Drutel A, Archambeaud F, Caron P. Selenium and the thyroid gland: more good news for clinicians. Clinical endocrinology 2013 Feb 1;78(2):155-64.
51. Betsy A, Binitha MP, Sarita S. Zinc deficiency associated with hypothyroidism: an overlooked cause of severe alopecia. International journal of trichology. 2013 Jan;5(1):40.

52. Dotevall G, Walan A. GASTRIC SECRETION OF ACID AND INTRINSIC FACTOR IN PATIENTS WITH HYPER-AND HYPOTHYROIDISM. Journal of Internal Medicine. 1969 Jan 12;186(1-6):529-33.
53. Ehrlich SD. Hypothyroidism [Internet]. Penn State Hershey Medical Center. American Accreditation HealthCare Commission ; Available from: http://pennstatehershey.adam.com/content.aspx?productId=107&pid=33&gid=000093#Supporting Research
54. Fatty Acids And The Role They Play In Thyroid Health [Internet]. Natural Endocrine Solutions. Available from: http://www.naturalendocrinesolutions.com/archives/fatty-acids-and-the-role-they-play-in-thyroid-health/
55. McMillan M, Spinks EA, Fenwick GR. Preliminary observations on the effect of dietary brussels sprouts on thyroid function. Human toxicology. 1986 Jan;5(1):15-9.
56. Chu M, Seltzer TF. Myxedema coma induced by ingestion of raw bok choy. New England Journal of Medicine. 2010 May 20;362(20):1945-6.
57. http://www.who.int/elena/titles/iodine_pregnancy/en/
58. van Zuuren EJ, Albusta AY, Fedorowicz Z, Carter B, Pijl H. Selenium supplementation

for Hashimoto's thyroiditis. The Cochrane Library. 2013 Jan 1.
59. Kandhro GA, Kazi TG, Afridi HI, Kazi N, Baig JA, Arain MB, Shah AQ, Sarfraz RA, Jamali MK, Syed N. Effect of zinc supplementation on the zinc level in serum and urine and their relation to thyroid hormone profile in male and female goitrous patients. Clinical Nutrition. 2009 Apr 1;28(2):162-8.
60. Wang YP, Lin HP, Chen HM, Kuo YS, Lang MJ, Sun A. Hemoglobin, iron, and vitamin B12 deficiencies and high blood homocysteine levels in patients with anti-thyroid autoantibodies. Journal of the Formosan Medical Association. 2014 Mar 1;113(3):155-60.
61. Stojanovich L. Stress and autoimmunity. Autoimmunity reviews. 2010 Mar 1;9(5):A271-6.
62. Wansink B, Van Ittersum K, Painter JE. Ice cream illusions: bowls, spoons, and self-served portion sizes. American journal of preventive medicine. 2006 Sep 1;31(3):240-3.
63. Dennis EA, Dengo AL, Comber DL, Flack KD, Savla J, Davy KP, Davy BM. Water consumption increases weight loss during a hypocaloric diet intervention in middle-aged and older adults. Obesity. 2010 Feb 1;18(2):300-7.
64. Zorrilla LM, Gibson EK, Jeffay SC, Crofton KM, Setzer WR, Cooper RL, Stoker

TE. The effects of triclosan on puberty and thyroid hormones in male Wistar rats. Toxicological Sciences. 2008 Oct 21;107(1):56-64.
65. Goldner WS, Sandler DP, Yu F, Hoppin JA, Kamel F, LeVan TD. Pesticide use and thyroid disease among women in the Agricultural Health Study. American journal of epidemiology. 2010 Jan 8;171(4):455-64.
66. Soldin OP, O'Mara DM, Aschner M. Thyroid hormones and methylmercury toxicity. Biological trace element research. 2008 Dec 1;126(1-3):1.
67. American Thyroid Association and American Association of Clinical Endocrinologists Taskforce on Hyperthyroidism and Other Causes of Thyrotoxicosis, Bahn RS, Burch HB, Cooper DS, Garber JR, Greenlee MC, Klein I, Laurberg P, McDougall IR, Montori VM, Rivkees SA. Hyperthyroidism and other causes of thyrotoxicosis: management guidelines of the American Thyroid Association and American Association of Clinical Endocrinologists. Thyroid. 2011 Jun 1;21(6):593-646.
68. Hyperthyroidism (Overactive Thyroid) [Internet]. The National Institute of Diabetes and Digestive and Kidney Diseases. NIH; Available from: https://www.niddk.nih.gov/health-

information/endocrine-diseases/hyperthyroidism
69. Hyperthyroidism (Overactive Thyroid) [Internet]. The National Institute of Diabetes and Digestive and Kidney Diseases. NIH; Available from: https://www.niddk.nih.gov/health-information/endocrine-diseases/hyperthyroidism
70. Devereaux D, Tewelde SZ. Hyperthyroidism and thyrotoxicosis. Emergency Medicine Clinics. 2014 May 1;32(2):277-92.
71. Ginsberg J. Diagnosis and management of Graves' disease. Canadian Medical Association Journal. 2003 Mar 4;168(5):575-85.
72. Beckett G, MacKenzie F. Thyroid guidelines-are thyroid-stimulating hormone assays fit for purpose?. Annals of clinical biochemistry. 2007 May 1;44(3):203-8.
73. Park HM. 123I: almost a designer radioiodine for thyroid scanning. Journal of Nuclear Medicine. 2002 Jan 1;43(1):77-8
74. Eber o, Buchinger w, Lindner w, Lind rath pe, Klima g, Langsteger w, Kõltringer p. The effect of d-versus l-propranolol in the treatment of hyperthyroidism. Clinical endocrinology. 1990 Mar 1;32(3):363-72.
75. Soley MH, Foreman N. Radioiodine therapy in graves'disease. The Journal of

clinical investigation. 1949 Nov 1;28(6):1367-74.
76. Fumarola A, Di Fiore A, Dainelli M, Grani G, Calvanese A. Medical treatment of hyperthyroidism: state of the art. Experimental and clinical endocrinology & diabetes. 2010 Nov 1;118(10):678.
77. Müssig K, Thamer C, Bares R, Lipp HP, Häring HU, Gallwitz B. Iodine-Induced Thyrotoxicosis After Ingestion of Kelp-Containing Tea. Journal of general internal medicine. 2006 Jun 1;21(6).
78. Di Matola T, Zeppa P, Gasperi M, Vitale M. Thyroid dysfunction following a kelp-containing marketed diet. BMJ case reports. 2014 Oct 29;2014:bcr2014206330.
79. Ch'ng CL, Jones MK, Kingham JG. Celiac disease and autoimmune thyroid disease. Clinical medicine & research. 2007 Oct 1;5(3):184-92.
80. Hwang IK, Kim SH, Lee U, Chin SO, Rhee SY, Oh S, Woo JT, Kim SW, Kim YS, Chon S. Celiac Disease in a predisposed subject (HLA-DQ2. 5) with coexisting Graves' disease. Endocrinology and Metabolism. 2015 Mar 1;30(1):105-9.
81. Joshi AS, Varthakavi PK, Bhagwat NM, Thiruvengadam NR. Graves' disease and coeliac disease: screening and treatment dilemmas. BMJ case reports. 2014 Oct 23;2014:bcr2013201386.

82. Ch'ng CL, Biswas M, Benton A, Jones MK, Kingham JG. Prospective screening for coeliac disease in patients with Graves' hyperthyroidism using anti-gliadin and tissue transglutaminase antibodies. Clinical endocrinology. 2005 Mar 1;62(3):303-6.
83. Mankaï A, Chadli-Chaieb M, Saad F, Ghedira-Besbes L, Ouertani M, Sfar H, Limem M, Abdessalem MB, Jeddi M, Chaieb L, Ghedira I. Screening for celiac disease in Tunisian patients with Graves' disease using anti-endomysium and anti-tissue transglutaminase antibodies. Gastroentérologie clinique et biologique. 2006 Aug 1;30(8-9):961-4.
84. Ventura A, Neri E, Ughi C, Leopaldi A, Città A, Not T. Gluten-dependent diabetes-related and thyroid-related autoantibodies in patients with celiac disease. The Journal of pediatrics. 2000 Aug 1;137(2):263-5.
85. Doerge DR, Sheehan DM. Goitrogenic and estrogenic activity of soy isoflavones. Environmental health perspectives. 2002 Jun;110(Suppl 3):349.
86. Cordle CT. Soy protein allergy: incidence and relative severity. The Journal of nutrition. 2004 May 1;134(5):1213S-9S.
87. Vojdani A, Erde J. Regulatory T cells, a potent immunoregulatory target for CAM researchers: the ultimate antagonist (I).

Evidence-Based Complementary and Alternative Medicine. 2006;3(1):25-30.
88. Li X, Wang G, Lu Z, Chen M, Tan J, Fang X. Serum 25-hydroxyvitamin D predict prognosis in radioiodine therapy of Graves' disease. Journal of endocrinological investigation. 2015 Jul 1;38(7):753-9.
89. Thyroid Function Tests [Internet]. Military Obstetrics & Gynecology. The Brookside Associates; Available from: http://www.brooksidepress.org/Products/Military_OBGYN/Lab/ThyroidFunctionTests.htm
90. Van der Watt G, Haarburger D, Berman P. Euthyroid patient with elevated serum free thyroxine. Clinical chemistry. 2008 Jul 1;54(7):1239-41.
91. Thyroid Function Tests [Internet]. Military Obstetrics & Gynecology. The Brookside Associates; Available from: http://www.brooksidepress.org/Products/Military_OBGYN/Lab/ThyroidFunctionTests.htm
92. Sinclair D. Thyroid antibodies: which, why, when and who?. Expert review of clinical immunology. 2006 Sep 1;2(5):665-9.
93. Moncayo H, Dapunt O, Moncayo R. Diagnostic accuracy of basal TSH determinations based on the intravenous TRH stimulation test: an evaluation of 2570 tests and comparison with the literature. BMC endocrine disorders. 2007 Dec;7(1):5.

94. Radioactive Iodine [Internet]. American Thyroid Association. Available from: https://www.thyroid.org/radioactive-iodine/

Disclaimer

The information contained in **"Healing Thyroid - Why You Still Have Thyroid Issues And How To Fix Them"** and its components, is meant to serve as a comprehensive collection of strategies that the author of this eBook has done research about. Summaries, strategies, tips and tricks are only recommendations by the author, and reading this eBook will not guarantee that one's results will exactly mirror the author's results.

The author of this Ebook has made all reasonable efforts to provide current and accurate information for the readers of this eBook. The author and its associates will not be held liable for any unintentional errors or omissions that may be found.

The material in the Ebook may include information by third parties. Third party materials comprise of opinions expressed by their owners. As such, the author of this eBook does not assume responsibility or liability for any third party material or opinions.

The publication of third party material does not constitute the author's guarantee of any information, products, services, or opinions contained within third party material. Use of third party material does not guarantee that your results will mirror our results. Publication of such third party material is simply a recommendation and expression of the author's own opinion of that material.

Whether because of the progression of the Internet, or the unforeseen changes in company policy and editorial submission guidelines, what is stated as fact at the time of this writing may become outdated or inapplicable later.

This Ebook is copyright ©2018 by **Neal Brown** with all rights reserved. It is illegal to redistribute, copy, or create derivative works from this Ebook whole or in parts. No parts of this report may be reproduced or retransmitted in any forms whatsoever without the written expressed and signed permission from the author.